"We didn't inherit the land from our fathers. We are borrowing it from our children." –

Amish Belief

ACKNOWLEDGEMENTS

This book is the culmination of many years of experience, some of which was the exciting pursuit of scientific fact and some was based on the pain of watching a loved one suffer. It is a journey of tremendous peaks and valleys but one thing is certain, this roller coaster ride was not boring. Through it all, I have met some incredible people who have made this a work of love and given me the thirst for knowledge which made it possible.

To my parents Frank and Anna who taught me right from wrong, who made sacrifices to come to the United States so my brother and I could have a chance to become something after the devastation of World War II Germany. You gave up so much for us that I can never repay you and will make sure my children will carry on your legacy and lessons for generations to come.

To the person who first showed me the excitement that health and nutrition could bring to an inquisitive mind, Alex, my brother. Thanks for making me leave New York when you did and exposing me to what was out there. Our time working together was short but it started me on my way. Whenever we get together now a days, I never cease to be amazed at how excited we still are about what we do after all these years.

My mentor of many years, John Kitkoski, I owe so much of my determination for the truth in science to you. May you have found the peace you so often sought for, my friend. Your mind worked at hyper speed but it was a just and determined brain nonetheless. You taught me to accept nothing at face value. Question everything but remember anything is possible as long as it remains true to science.

My business partner and long-time friend Tim Gary, one of the most honest human beings I have had the pleasure to have met. I wouldn't have wanted to start Carbon Based Corporation (nor could I have) without your incredible skills as a programmer and person extraordinaire. Without that vehicle, none of this would have been possible.

Robert Crayhon. I consider myself so lucky to have met a friend like you. Your soul is so good and caring I heeded your demand that I put this book together. Thanks for the numerous kicks in the butt; I needed it.

All of this would have no meaning if not for my "other" family. Pete and Nancy, my in-laws, you have been so supportive of me. Words cannot express you how much I appreciate it. Your support when the chips were down was incredible.

Hillary, my wife, I still don't know how you put up with me. You have been my rock, my friend and the person who supported me when others tried to steal my work while our oldest child was suffering through her health challenges. You never gave up on me; thanks.

To my wonderful daughter Anika, your happy demeanor and loving nature makes Daddy's day go by with a smile.

Last but not least, my brave little girl Tasya. What you went through over these past many years would have crippled lesser people. Your firmly held belief that in spite of all that has transpired, your father would find a way to make you better. This faith in me has driven me to heights which I could not have reached without you; you are an inspiration to me that has touched me to my very soul.

CONTENTS

INTRODUCTION

"In my writing I am acting as a map maker, an explorer of psychic... a cosmonaut of inner space, and I see no point in exploring areas that have already been thoroughly surveyed."

William Burroughs

"The way a child discovers the world constantly replicates the way science began. You start to notice what's around you, and you get very curious about how things work. How things interrelate. It's as simple as seeing a bug that intrigues you. You want to know where it goes at night; who its friends are; what it eats."

David Cronenberg

"If we make a couple of discoveries here and there we need not believe things will go on like this for ever.... Just as we hit water when we dig in the earth, so we discover the incomprehensible sooner or later."

G. C. Lichtenberg

"Hurray, you finally got it, Mark!" my dear friend and colleague Dr. Ann McCombs, an osteopath based in Bellevue, Washington exclaimed. I felt slightly embarrassed as I should have "gotten" it a long time ago, but I need convincing and good scientific validation before I buy into any theories. Things also have to make sense in the grand scheme of things as in my mind, nothing works in a vacuum.

So what was it that I finally understood after being in the laboratory interpretation and health education business since 1983? What was it that would change my world and help me teach people about an issue that will not only have ramifications in their lives today, but for their children and the lives of billions of people yet to be born?

TOXICITY.

Simple, yet so complex, the concept of toxicity is one that cannot be overstated by any stretch of the imagination. It is my belief that it is at the core of every health issue we face in the world today. It transcends health having enormous consequences in the arena of social interactions, behavior, politics, both national and global, as well as being involved in the very survival of all living species on the big blue marble we call Earth.

Mark, what a melodramatic introduction but don't you think you've gone a little overboard with your comments?

I only wish that was true. The frightening fact is that I may be far too reserved with my observations. As you will see in this book the facts are more disturbing than you can imagine.

According to an interview on CNN.com, Dr. Leo Trasande stated "We are in an epidemic of environmentally mediated disease among American children today," he said. "Rates of asthma, childhood cancers, birth defects and developmental disorders have exponentially increased, and it can't be explained by changes in the human genome. So what has changed? All the chemicals we're being exposed to."

When I start my lectures, I compare myself and my talks to a Stephen King novel being turned into a movie by Wes Craven. They are scary not by design but they turn out to be because the truth in this case is frightening. A note left behind on a table at a one-day seminar where I spoke at with Robert Crayhon and Dr. Dietrich Klinghardt, commented that the attendee was glad they wouldn't be alive to see the havoc caused by the issues I brought up. The author of the note also commented at how scary my lecture was.

As you shall see in Section 2 of this book, the writer of the comment is alive to see the havoc. It is already upon us and each and every one of us is suffering through the greatest experiment that has ever been undertaken in human history; an experiment that if not controlled soon may have dire consequences.

This book though is not all doom and gloom. It is one of hope. It is a book that I believe will provide you the tools to make a difference in your own lives as well as the life of loved ones and the rest of humanity. You are embarking on a tour of our world written by an optimistic realist. Despite what I have seen in my almost 50 years of life, I still think that there is not only hope of survival but hope of creating a better environment for our children to live in, one that we will be proud of when our time is up. It is also a book to make each of our days better, healthier, and happier.

This book is divided into four sections. Each one of the sections could have been a book unto itself but I really felt deep down that it needed to be put together to paint a complete picture of the world as I see it.

Section 1: Tasya's Story. My lovely daughter Tasya, born in 1996, is in my opinion and many others who know her, one of the bravest people around. A beautiful, warm-hearted child who has had the misfortune of dealing with a neurological disorder that at times was life threatening – epilepsy. My mother Anna, who is one heck of a brave person herself having survived the horrors of Europe during World War II, when seeing my daughter have one of her drop (atonic) seizures said, "My health problems don't seem so bad, I need to stop complaining about what I'm going through and be like my grandchild." This from a woman who has suffered triple bypass surgery, breast cancer, colon cancer, and back surgery in the past fifteen years.

This segment of the book was the hardest to write. It was as emotional of a time as anyone could imagine. What my wife Hillary and I went through would have torn many couples apart, yet it made both of us stronger and closer than we could have ever imagined. What Tasya went through is the story of legends. As I sit here writing this tears well up in my eyes knowing of what she went through with her chin up and a smile on her face. I truly hope her story will inspire you as it did me and many others around her.

Next is: Our Toxic World. This part of the book is where I really unload on the reader and hopefully put fear into your minds and souls. It is a sobering section that begins with a history of how we intoxicate our environment. I use the word intoxicate here because what we have done is similar to what happens to a drunk person, we have lost the ability to make rational decisions because of the sheer quantity of toxins we have dumped into ourselves. We don't know when to stop because we have become addicted to the short term pleasures these toxins have seemingly brought into our lives. One chapter is devoted into defining what a toxin is, and it is a lot broader of a definition than you think. I then take you on a tour of todays broken down medical industry, the toxic sludge makers, and the economic ramifications of our downward environmental spiral and the implications that our toxic ecosystem will have on our health as well as the health of many generations to come.

To typify how toxicity affects us daily, I will follow a typical morning of two couples, both of whom try to live "healthy" lives. One couple does a great job and the other is more like everyone else, getting bombarded by toxins from places that they never would have imagined. Looking in the mirror, you will never give you the same view the world around you the same way ever again.

Thirdly, How to Achieve Victory Over a Toxic World. As my good friend Robert Crayhon put it, "Mark, you've got to give people hope otherwise they'll walk away being pretty darned depressed." Advice well heeded my friend. As I like to put it, this is my Disney part of the book. This is where heroes abound and I deliver the tools you need to win the battle against our polluted environment.

This scientifically researched and clinically relevant book will give you the means to detoxify yourself, along with the map of the roads to achieving optimal health. One has to remember as author Hannah Green once said, "Health is not simply the absence of sickness." We as a society have accepted a level of "health" that is, in my opinion, unacceptable. Chronic illness is tolerated when it shouldn't be. Health is vibrancy. Health is energy and enthusiasm. Health is vitality. It is not just surviving another day, no it is *thriving* in the day. Looking forward to everyday not as though it will be your last but as though it is the first day all over again.

One focus of this section will be in differentiating fact from fiction. My favorite President, Abraham Lincoln was asked "If a horse's tail is called a leg, how many legs does a horse have?" "Four." Abe replied, "Calling a horse's tail a leg does not make it a leg." All too often in the world of health people try to claim that their horse's tail (I'm using nice words here) is a leg when in reality it isn't. I will attempt to steer the reader clear of the many horse's **cough, cough ** tails out there.

Since my vocation according to my Rotary Blue Badge is Laboratory Interpretations, no book by me would be complete without in-depth discussions of these valuable tools. My work at Carbon Based Corporation and the development of the CellMate Reports™ now known as LabAssist™ as well as being the head of product development at Knowledge Through Solutions (since merged into Crayhon Research) has provided me with insights that I will share with you. These chapters are geared towards both the health care practitioner and the patient. I hope my 20+ years in the field and my enthusiasm will excite you as much as it has me.

I will also discuss the tools of the trade, all the tools and how to use them which is great, but you need to know where to get them. We need to know what the best tools are and which ones to be avoided as well. This is the section that will hopefully be the one you will wear out the fastest as I hope you go back to this over and over in an ongoing endeavor to achieve victory over our toxic world.

While the Internet is a great vehicle in which to find information it is also a bastion of misinformation, misguided advice, myths, legends, and downright lies. I will send you packing for a trip around the world without leaving the comfort of your home to the best sites, with the best information, and let you learn more than I could ever teach you in this book.

Another section will introduce you to companies that sell what I feel are the best supplements available. Being actively involved in this end of the alternative health world gives me an insight few outsiders have and it will allow me to guide you towards the best of the best out there and hopefully save you time and money as well.

While I think my book should be on everyone's book shelf and in every library, it doesn't cover every topic I'd like to. If it tried to, I'd still be writing it and the Reno Centennial Sunset Rotary Club members (inside joke) would be still bugging me to get this book done. So, in this chapter you can find a number of books I've read and used over the years that will provide you with more detailed information on many of the topics I will go over here.

My friend Robert once told me in the context of speakers and the conferences he puts together, "If there is one thing you shouldn't do as a speaker is bore people." I sincerely hope that this book doesn't bore but excites, frightens, and inspires you. So, strap yourselves in and get ready for a spellbinding trip through the world you and I live in.

PART I

1. A Little Background

At a conference put on by Dr. Dietrich Klinghardt, an internationally renowned physician and scientist, I was introduced by him as being famous for three things. One was being the brother of noted researcher Alexander Schauss. This, he suggested, hints at a possible genetic predisposition for research in the field. Secondly, he said that another claim of fame I had was spending nine plus years mentoring under the brilliant scientist John Kitkoski in Spokane, Washington. Thirdly, I am known for developing a unique methodology for interpreting laboratory test results that has revolutionized the way we look at data.

My initial reaction was to be somewhat honored but I thought of two other things I would rather be known for, things that are far more important. The first and most obvious to me is that I am a father who would not accept "we don't know" for an answer when it came to my daughter's health. The other reason for fame is being a bluntly honest person, who tells it like is and that I will never, ever claim to have all the answers. It is my deep seated belief that as soon as you think you have "the" answer, you don't and you run the risk of putting barricades in front of your continued search for answers to the question of achieving optimal health.

So, how did I start on my lifetime journey?

I first started looking at "alternative" medicine back in 1983 while working for my brother, Dr. Alexander Schauss, the President of the American Institute for Biomedical Research in Tacoma, Washington. Alex's work includes the pioneering book, "*Diet, Crime and Delinquency*" which proposed a theory that there was a link between your behavior and what you ate. His library was a treasure trove of information that I immersed myself in, working from 8:00 am to midnight trying to learn as much as possible.

After my 1½ year stint with Alex, I was ready to move on and try new and innovative things. My next association was with a person who would change the way I thought about everything in life, "Crazy" John.

John Kitkoski was considered a brilliant madman, someone who could ramble on for days about everything under the sun. He also had a way of teaching that was borne of the school of hardest knocks. While working with and for him, you understood quickly that the request to "hold these two wires and put your foot in this bucket of water" was often times an invitation to a shocking experience but was also meant to teach you something you would never forget.

Kitkoski, as we called him, was a self-proclaimed physicist with a distinct focus on nutrition. He had almost 500 college credits to his name but no degree. He had read the entire medical library at the local hospital while recovering from a broken neck and back. His life was thinking of how to make things better and more logical.

After working with him at his company, Life Balances, one important comment kept resonating in my head..... "If the concept you're working on breaks laws of chemistry or physics, abandon it. Move on."

He put a couple of other important thoughts into my head that has guided my way of thinking since. Here are some of the most important and their meanings:

You can't carry two tons of manure in a one ton truck.
If you try to carry around toxins in your body, you're eventually going to be unable to continue operating efficiently and something major is going to break down.

You can't run a Cadillac on a Volkswagen diet.
Human beings need to be fed like a high class machine. You need to make sure that you feed yourself high quality foods and drinks, not junk foods and sugar rich drinks.

If it sounds too good to be true, it is.
Now I know this is a common saying but he emphatically emphasized it. With it came a caveat, don't necessarily throw out an idea you don't like, but look at it critically and honestly lest you miss out on a great discovery.

Another thing that he kept reminding me about was that while looking at a problem, take the panoramic view first before you get into the details. Too often scientists, and especially health care practitioners, look at the leaf in the forest, rightly determine that it's sick, and try to dissect it trying to find out what metabolic abnormalities are afoot causing the leaf to be unhealthy. Some will even put on multi-day seminars discussing the biochemical pathways that are at the root of the leaf's demise and ill fortunes. Unfortunately, they fail to see that the real reason the leaf is sick and brown is that the forest is on fire. Sometimes health care practitioners can get caught up in the minutia and fail to see the bigger picture, like baseline electrolyte balance, amino acid balance, and nutrient competency.

John also stressed that you have to remember the concept that no nutrient, medication, food, or substance of any kind acts like the Lone Ranger. What you take in has a ripple effect and that just because there is an initial good effect does not mean everything related to that item is good. His lesson here was to make sure that everyone always understands that when you take something, reactions cause other reactions. Just because water flushes out toxins, this does not mean that it will avoid flushing out nutrients too. Too many people give things like water a brain, as though it would know the difference between something bad and something good.

America is the land of instant pudding. One of our worst attributes is that we are wholly unwilling to take time to do something. We only want to do things that give us instant gratification. Diets have to work now! What do you mean I have to change my lifestyle forever? Impatience equals failure. Ever hear of the story of the turtle and the hare?

Can't you give me a pill to make it all better, bigger, stronger, and smarter? I can't (read won't) give up my 12 pack of beer every night. It's the only way I can get to sleep. Cigarettes? They're impossible to quit. Just give me something to tide me over won't ya? No, we can't and even if we do, it won't solve anything. America's greatest generation gave birth to America's laziest generation.

Time is a nutrient. Use it wisely, but don't forget to add it to the health equation. NUTRIENTS WILL NOT RESOLVE YOUR HEALTH ISSUES IMMEDIATELY! They take time to act out their entire play. Think of that process. Also, remember the concept of the Lone Ranger. Since they do not work alone, their reactions cannot happen instantaneously. Allow nutrient interactions to happen. Be patient.

Be skeptical and apply the previous concepts to your decisions about what is real and what isn't. When someone says "Product XYZ will cure whatever you have and you'll get results right away" run to the nearest exit, and run like hell. No one has "the answer".

Ptolemy, in his work the *Almagest*, wrote that the earth was at the center of the universe and everything circled it in concentric globes. This theory ruled as the truth until a man named Copernicus came around and developed a new truth that had the sun at the center with the earth circling it. This became the new truth in its time until Johannes Kepler took Tycho Brahe's information and developed a new theory which changed the way we looked at our world until Sir Isaac Newton stood on "the shoulder of giants" and revolutionized things yet again. That is, until a small man with wild hair named Albert Einstein changed things yet once more.

Each person had an answer but not "the answer". They all had an opinion about what was right, and how things worked. Time and new findings change what we know regularly. Anyone who claims to have found "the answer" should be avoided or at least looked upon with great skepticism. If not, the cost will be more expensive than you are ready to deal with. The cost may include your life or the life of the person you are treating.

My doctorate is in business, not medicine, not biochemistry or any other health related field. What I have learned is how to see a problem in a unique way. I have not been prejudiced by the dogma of institutional learning yet I have been subjected to the rigor education brings which is meticulous thought, reasoning, and questioning. As you shall also find, I am guided by the force of family and the need to save one of the most precious jewels I have ever come upon, my daughter Tasya.

My background allows me to be subjective, opinionated, and critical yet forces me to look at things with a passion only a parent can have. If what you are looking for is honesty and not the "company line", count yourself lucky. This is what I hope you will find in this book.

2. TASYA'S STORY

"There are only two or three human stories, and they go on repeating themselves as fiercely as if they had never happened before."

Willa Cather

"Listen little Elia: draw your chair up close to the edge of the precipice and I'll tell you a story."

F. Scott Fitzgerald

"The book which the reader now holds in his hands, from one end to the other, as a whole and in its details, whatever gaps, exceptions, or weaknesses it may contain, treats of the advance from evil to good; from injustice to justice, from falsity to truth, from darkness to daylight, from blind appetite to conscience, from decay to life, from bestiality to duty, from Hell to Heaven, from limbo to God. Matter itself is the starting-point, and the point of arrival is the soul. Hydra at the beginning, an angel at the end."

Victor Hugo from Les Misérables.

"Daddy, I just fell on my butt." giggled my little three and a half year old as I came home from work.

My wife Hillary seemed a bit concerned as it was a sudden fall backwards. I brushed it off as just a child's clumsiness and it didn't seem to have any effect on my daughter Tasya. Still, Hillary was a bit concerned, but that passed quickly.

We had been married four years now and we wanted to go out for our anniversary dinner. The babysitter was called and she was due at our house at about 6:00 pm. It was a few weeks later than the actual date we were married but we were so busy with our businesses at the time. Hillary and I were thrilled nonetheless that we were going to have a few hours alone.

Little did we know that we were about to embark on one of the most incredible and horrifying journeys of our lives. One fraught with fear, anger, frustration, exaltation, and a motive to devote our lives to something we were singularly blessed with, the ability to share the resources we had to help fight a frightening condition known as epilepsy.

It was somewhere around 5:45 pm and we were awaiting the arrival of the babysitter. Tasya was playing downstairs in her room, down the hall from our bedroom. I was, as usual, dressed and ready before my wife, so I started down the hall, ready to go upstairs to have a glass of wine when I saw something that scared me to my very core. My daughter, the absolute light of my life, was on the floor shaking and convulsing violently.

Hillary was on the phone with her mom Nancy, when I screamed at her to hang-up and call 911. I remember the expression on her face, sheer horror. Something was happening to her baby she couldn't fathom. She yelled to her mom that she had to go because something terrible was happening to Tasya. She immediately called 911.

Our town, where we lived at the time, is a small, but beautiful spot on the north shore of Lake Tahoe, a pristine environment (or so we thought), safe and quiet, friends everywhere. Incline Village, Nevada is the kind of town most people would love to live in. We were happy to raise our daughter in such a peaceful place. Little did we know that the closeness of the fire department and paramedics would be just as important to us.

Help was on its way as emergency services are within minutes of our home. Tasya continued seizing, while I was helplessly trying to get her to relax, not knowing what was going on. We could hear the paramedics and fire department coming in the background but what was only 2-3 minutes seemed like a lifetime.

Briefly I thought that she was choking on something as I couldn't imagine that somehow she was having an epileptic seizure. I tried to perform the Heimlich maneuver to dislodge whatever it was that was choking her. Not being well versed in what to do when a person is having an epileptic fit, I put my finger in her mouth so she wouldn't bite her tongue (don't do that, I later found out it was the wrong thing to do).

We kept calling to her, begging her to wake up and make this just a nightmare that would go away quickly. As the sirens got closer and the 911 operator tried her best to keep us calm, Tasya's spasms began to abate.

Just as the paramedics arrived, the happiest sound a father or mother could ever hear in a time like this echoed through the halls; a scream. I never thought that a yell like hers could ever sound so thrilling, but it did. She cried because she didn't know what had happened to her. Her face of fear and panic is something I will never forget. She was scared of all the people around her. She wanted her mommy.

One of the paramedics was someone we knew, but at the time I couldn't tell and I didn't care. All I cared about was how my baby was doing. Nothing else mattered in the world, nor would it for the next few years.

Even though she seemed okay, the recommendation was to take her to the hospital to be sure that nothing else was going to happen. The babysitter arrived, obviously stunned to see what was going on. We sadly informed her that she probably wasn't going to be needed tonight, or as we later realized, not for a long, long time.

Pete and Nancy, my in-laws, raced in through the downstairs door frantically wondering what had happened. Luckily for us, they also live just a few minutes away from us. The two of them were to be our Rocks of Gibraltar as we began to unravel the mystery that surrounded our child's epilepsy. They followed Hillary and me as we drove Tasya to the hospital in Truckee to start her on a series of tests that were to become part of her life for the next few months.

When we reached the hospital, the doctor and nurses on staff took the three of us into the emergency room and began to interview us.

'What happened', 'Has she ever had a seizure before', 'Do any of her relatives have a history of epilepsy?'

The answers were: "We don't know," "Not that we've ever seen," and "No."

They told us that the first thing that they were going to do is draw blood to run a series of tests to see what is going on. As they tried to explain what the blood test is going to tell them, I explained that I probably could teach them what they were looking for as I was the President of a company that did blood test interpretations for health care practitioners.

I knew in my heart already, that I was going to use that knowledge to help Tasya. What I didn't know was how many others were going to be helped by what I found. It was also going to show me what true friends were really like.

The next test they wanted to run was a CT scan. After the trauma of the blood draw, which Tasya definitely did not like (very vocal about her opinion of needles), I was worried that she wouldn't stay still for the scan. Nothing could be further from the truth. As we were to see in the coming months, she was determined to allow us to find out what was happening to her so she "could get better".

As the doctor explained, the CT scan was merely being done to rule out tumors or gross abnormalities in the brain.

Horrible thoughts came into my mind, "What if there is something there?" "How would we handle it if there really was one?"

The thoughts were heightened as we remembered that another little girl in our town had a cancerous brain tumor and she was only a year older than our baby. Unfortunately, she didn't survive very much longer.

Tasya was a trooper though, she called the scanner a "big doughnut" and she was as still as can be. If only adults could be as brave as her. It's what held me up for the next few months. Dad had to be as brave as his little girl.

The CT scan came back negative, which was a great relief to both Hillary and me. The blood test, while not complete gave me some clues as to what was happening biochemically and years later they were at the core of our goal to help her get better. My arrogance, which was to pop up way too many times, led me to believe that I would be able to find the answers quickly as I was smart enough to do it by sheer brute intellectual force. The next six and a half years were to prove otherwise and teach me a big lesson in humility.

Between those first days and today, Tasya has had eleven waking grand mal seizures. The smallest was about four minutes and the longest was around six hours. We lost count of the number of nocturnal seizures she's had as she would have one almost every morning before awakening for years. The drop seizures, where her body jerks violently forward, which she has had from the age of five on, probably number in the thousands. And the twitches and shakes are too numerous to imagine. Those are numbers previously used by Carl Sagan in his discussions on the number of stars in the sky on his show *Cosmos*.

Things were looking bleak for Tasya, yet through it all, she somehow kept up her spirits. Seizure after seizure, especially the petite mals, which she knew were coming, were making her miserable.

Then one day she looked at me and uttered words only a child could say, yet it was a sentence that is forever burned in my memory as the most painful, yet challenging moment of my life:

"Daddy, why can't you fix me?"

Never in my life did words ever cut as deep into my soul as those six words did. She knew that I devoted my life to helping people with medical problems and that I hadn't been there for her. Looking at her with tear soaked eyes she uttered another few words that at once invigorated me and also made me determined to find an answer to her disorder:

"But Daddy, I know you will make me better soon."

I never looked back and never felt sorry for myself again. At that instant, I knew that I had to solve my daughter's seizure mystery.

She had just gone through a horrific forty-five minute seizure that day some six weeks into her ordeal and was pretty worn but she wanted to see her grandparents. We had them over for dinner, all of us quiet and somber but Tasya would have none of that. She wanted to have stories read to her, listen to songs and have fun. Tasya had no time for pity and sadness.

Maybe it was because of her youthful innocence and maybe it was her refusal to succumb to our somber nature. I suspect it was because she was her Mom's daughter. Stubborn and head strong, unwilling to give up, she always wanted to climb that next mountain despite the discomfort.

But through it all, her smiles, hopefulness, and resolute nature continue to amaze and inspire me. So much so that if any of you ever meet me and hear me complaining about any aches and pains, take a stick and whack me once or twice because whatever I'm going through is nothing compared to what she has had to endure in her brief life.

3. LIFE IN THE BEGINNING

"Although it is generally known, I think it's about time to announce that I was born at a very early age."

Groucho Marx

"My mother groan'd, my father wept,
Into the dangerous world I leapt;
Helpless, naked, piping loud,
Like a fiend hid in a cloud."

William Blake

"We are not what we are, nor do we treat or esteem each other for such, but for what we are capable of being."

Henry David Thoreau

Born on a snowy day on April 17, 1996, Anastasya Janine Schauss came into this world after my wife Hillary and I went though a thirty-six hour ordeal of back labor. Ok, so Hillary did 99% of the work and I was there merely to supply support. After thirty hours of attempting to try natural child birth complete with a Douala, Hillary decided to follow the suggestion of the nurse and have an epidural.

Six blissful hours later (according to my wife), Tasya decided to come out just as fast as she could, right now, no hesitation. The doctor scrambled to catch my little girl, begging Hillary to slow down (something that was no longer under her control it seemed). We should have known right then and there that Anastasya was going to do things on her own time frame and her way.

When I first saw her, my heart filled with a joy that is hard to put into words. Anyone who has witnessed the miracle of childbirth knows what I'm talking about. Although she was covered with a green slime, the male nurse cleaned her up and quickly sucked up what little meconium (an infant's first stool) had gotten into her mouth. The doctor then pronounced to all in the room that we had a healthy baby girl. Her Apgar score was 9s all around. Darn near perfect.

A peculiar patch of pigmented skin was wrapped around her left arm, shoulder and chest, but we were told not to worry about it. This was a mistake. We found out nine years later that there was a very definite link between her café au lait birth mark and her seizures.

As I describe later, during fetal development, the skin and brain develop from the same cells. The markings on her skin signify a relationship between the skin and brain development. No one knows why this happens and what to do about it. My belief is that it is at this time, Tasya and Hillary were exposed to a toxin. What it was, we will never know but research shows that there are critical periods during fetal brain development and that toxins can play a devastating role.

Holding this little bundle of life made me appreciate all that was good with the world. Little did I know that it would also show me some of the dark underbelly of science and medicine. It also made me painfully aware of those who would exploit other parent's misery and desperation to feed their need for money and ego gratification.

Carefully, I handed Tasya, as we had decided to call her, to my wife who for good reason, was still pretty out of it with the drugs and all having just given birth to a six pound six ounce girl. Tears flowed down my cheeks as I stared at mother and daughter snuggling together for the first time ever. I was so proud I wanted to tell the world, I was finally a father at the age of thirty seven!

Next up for the new parents was sleep, but not before our first argument with the head strong all-knowing (she was, just ask her) nurse.

She came in telling us we had to have a Hepatitis B vaccination right away as it is important to protect our child from this dreaded disease. I responded to her rather tersely that the chance of her getting Hep B at this point and for the next dozen plus years was the equivalent to getting hit by a bolt of lightening in the middle of the Mohave Desert during the dry season. In other words, the odds were ridiculously low.

Now I'm not one to blame vaccinations for all our children's ills, but darn it, a vaccination at six hours old? For something there is almost no chance of her contracting in the foreseeable future, especially at that age? Obviously, Tasya did not get a Hep B shot that day (or since). We firmly but convincingly made it clear that this was an event that was not going to happen today.

The good thing about our argument was that when our next child Anika was born at that same hospital, they did not offer that shot, they hadn't for six years since Tasya was born. They felt that the risk versus reward numbers were not high enough to warrant the shot at such an early age. It made me feel good to hear that. One small step for Tasya equaled many saved kids. Unfortunately, they reverted back to giving Hep B vaccinations to newborns just recently. Sad but true.

Tasya's first three years of life seemed pretty normal. She was fussy at times, a little colicky, but usually quite happy. Sometimes, she could cry for what seemed like an eternity although it was not very often. She was also one of the most hiccuppingest (I love that word) kids I had ever seen. Tasya would go into hiccupping fits for no reason. I later found out that this is not uncommon in epileptic children and may be a type of seizure.

Looking back, we probably should have noticed something, but in reality, she seemed just like any other kid. There were probably signs we should have wondered about but we just wanted to believe our child was going to be special and of course, healthy.

When Tasya was eighteen months, Hillary, her parents and I were sitting around our coffee table when Tasya came running, tripped, and hit the table with her forehead. While everyone was panicking to stop the bleeding, Dad calmly took care of the situation as he was an old hand at this, having done the same thing twice to himself in his youth. We took Tasya to the emergency room, a place she was someday to know all too well, where they stitched her up. We were told to watch over her after the accident so we kept her in bed with us that night. Nothing happened and she seemed no worse for the wear.

The years went on and we were so happy that our daughter was healthier than most other kids. She never seemed to get a cold, never had an earache, and slept like a log from early on. Our comfort, soon to be shattered, was helpful as we were in the midst of fighting a lawsuit brought on by our ex-partners (and one time best friends) who were trying to break me financially and emotionally so they could take all of my years of work as their own. Our stress levels were at an all time high, but our kid was healthy as could be, or so we thought.

We were so sure of how healthy Tasya was that we switched health insurance plans to save a few dollars. Much to our chagrin, the insurance company we chose was one that thought that an MRI and a CT scan were unnecessary after my child was diagnosed with epilepsy. Every time I hear their commercial touting their concern for the high cost of health insurance for small business owners and how they will save you money, I cringe. The change cost us upwards of $20,000 and saved us nothing.

All of that confidence in us being a healthy family made us yearn for a second child, but only after the stress of running our businesses subsided. So we put off these thoughts, as bringing a kid into such a rough situation wasn't right.

But still, Tasya was healthy, until that fateful October day when she had her first seizure.

About four days after her first seizure, with us hoping that it was only going to be a one time occurrence, we took Tasya out trick o' treating. Our first stop was the local fire station in Crystal Bay, Nevada where her best friend James's dad worked. She was dressed as Cinderella. She was my princess and she knew it.

While whirling around to show off her dress to the firefighters, she fell to the ground and went into another convulsion. The paramedics went right into action and got her on some oxygen. She came to about four minutes later panicked, and crying again.

Hillary looked at me and didn't have to say a word. I knew how shattered she felt. We began to understand that we were on a journey and not a short ride.

When we took her to our in-laws house to at least get some joy out of Halloween, our hearts sunk to the floor looking at our little girl who was so unsure of what was going on yet so desperate to enjoy her "candy day" like all the other children. I was so protective of her I couldn't leave her side.

Our next step was to see a pediatric neurologist. This was our first glimpse into the world of ego, conjecture, and arrogance. It was not going to be our last.

We went into the doctor's office hoping to get a clear answer into Tasya's epilepsy but instead we found a cold person who wanted us to just listen to her and not question anything she told us. She was an epileptologist and we were not. There was no team effort to help our kid. Do as you are told and nothing else.

Her diagnosis was generalized juvenile myoclonic epilepsy and the treatment was Depakote™, a drug also known as valproic acid. Nothing more, nothing less. Take it or leave it. When I asked about any nutritional supplements that might be helpful, I was looked at as though I had just announced that the moon was made of green cheese.

She went on to say that there was a chance that the diagnosis would add a progressive connotation to it which meant that things would get worse and that the prognosis was very poor if that were the case. The doctor tried, in her dour and cold way to bolster us by saying that it might not be progressive, but we knew deep down that it probably was although Hillary and I said nothing to each other about that.

After the diagnosis of epilepsy was given to us we sat in the car in stunned silence, knowing, but not wanting to admit that our child and our lives would never be the same. We felt devastated but I knew from the deepest reaches of my soul that somehow, someday, I would find an answer that would allow Tasya to live a normal and healthy life.

How do you admit that your child isn't normal, that she isn't like the other kids? As parents, we look at everything they do and marvel at their first word, their first step, when they get potty trained and we think 'our kid is special'. Somehow the neurologist made us feel that our kid was somehow defective. It was a brutal blow we were unwilling to accept.

From here, we went to the local Costco pharmacy to get her prescription filled and started her on Depakote™ sprinkles hoping that the seizures would stop and Tasya could go back to leading a normal life. This was not to be the case.

Thankfully, I had a number of medical advisors to my company that I was able to call upon for advice. Unfortunately, not many had ever dealt with a child with epilepsy. My first clue in helping my kid came from Dr. Richard Lord, a biochemist who works for a specialty lab in Atlanta, Georgia called MetaMetrix. He told me to look at amino acids, especially taurine.

I began to do research on the internet, spending hours reading every bit of information I could come up with. Sleep was a luxury that I had to grab sparingly as I was determined to find answers.

Hillary took Tasya to Children's Hospital in Seattle, Washington at the request of Tasya's Godfather Michael Levitz. Mike was a professor of Biostatistics at the University of Washington and someone I considered to be like family. His wife, Inesa, was a physician who was to help us with advice and emotional support. We wanted to get a second opinion but what we really wanted was a better diagnosis, one that would not be as severe and threatening. Unfortunately, that was not to be the case.

While I was searching for answers, Tasya had one seizure after another. Each grand mal was longer and more violent, shaking my girl harder and harder. Not only that but she couldn't handle sunlight peaking through the trees as the strobe effect caused her to convulse. We could not take short drives with her in the car unless she was wearing dark sunglasses which did not always work. We felt hopeless.

Still, we wanted Tasya to have some enjoyment in life in between her seizures. Whenever we could play with her, we did. One day in mid-October, we took her to the playground at the beach on the shores of Lake Tahoe so she could at least go on the swings and have a little fun and smile again.

Tasya laughed and giggled as she started going back and forth, strapped into the swing so we felt safer. All of a sudden, her eyes rolled back into her head and she began to convulse. We struggled to try to get her out of the swing as she continued to seize. Her body was so stiff we almost couldn't get her free. People were coming around asking if they could help. We finally got her loose of the seat but her seizure was not stopping.

Our house was four blocks away from the playground which is where our car was so I ran to the house as fast as I could and drove back as fast as I could. Calling for an ambulance and waiting wasn't an option as I figured I could get her to the hospital a lot faster. The other thought, which filled me with so much guilt, was that we needed to save some money as we knew our insurance was worthless and that the ambulance was another expense we could not bear.

It is the dream of every parent, regardless of their socio-economic background, to provide the best for their child. We yearn to make things better for them yet, at that moment, I felt like such a failure. I was so angry at so many people. It was something I had to let go of but it took years to accomplish.

Stress was the main problem I was putting on my child and wife, it was the last thing either of them needed. One of the most important steps in healing Tasya was to heal myself. I needed to work out my anger and above all take care of my child. Anyone who has a special needs child knows how hard that is. This is why so many marriages with autistic or epileptic children end in divorce.

When we got Tasya to the hospital, I was thrilled to see that Dr. Joe Ryan, a warm and caring physician, was attending the emergency room. He looked at her and asked how long had she been seizing. It had been twenty-five minutes, the longest one yet.

He tried to get a line into her tiny veins to get her on some Valium to stop the seizure. It wasn't working. Dr. Ryan looked almost panicked trying hard to do whatever he could do to stop the seizure. My wife and I felt that we were losing our child as we asked what the ramifications were of this long seizure and the reply was not positive.

"Brain damage is a distinct possibility if I can't stop it soon," was Dr. Ryan's reply.

Just then I asked him if I could try something, a technique I learned from an osteopath I met at a medical seminar. Dr. Ryan told me to do what I could since he was having no success in administering Valium.

I pushed on her neck, near the carotid artery, massaging the muscle and lo and behold her seizure just stopped. Did the manipulation do it? I cannot definitively say yes or no but her seizure did come to an end and that was all that mattered.

Hillary and I were winded and wiped out. Our emotions had taken a high speed roller coaster ride and all we wanted was to get our baby home. What we did not realize was that this was to be the worst seizure she was to have for many years to come.

After the horrific events of the day, we cocooned her that evening, holding her and hugging her until she had had enough. She was squirming around not wanting to be over protected anymore but we had a hard time letting go. She wanted to be independent and free and all we wanted was to protect her.

Our only thought was, "When would this all stop?"

During the time between seizure number two at the fire station and the long seizure at the park, we were starting to get an array of nutrients into her, most of which we got from our good friends at Kirkman Labs in Portland, Oregon (see resources). They had a variety of nutrients that were in a liquid or powder form, making them easier for Tasya to swallow. We also gave her methylcobalamin, a very absorbable form of vitamin B12, which came as a nasal spray.

While my girl was not thrilled with the idea, she was willing to do anything to help control the seizures. Of course, all the while we were giving her Depakote™ sprinkles in apple sauce, about the only way she would take it, per the neurologist's orders.

When we started adding taurine, a neuroinhibitory (calmative) amino acid to Tasya's regime, which we put into the apple sauce as well, things took a turn for the better. She no longer was shuddering when we passed through lights, her nocturnal seizures were lessening in severity, and she seemed clearer and not as "drugged out" as before. We were also getting some liquid magnesium into her which is considered quite beneficial due to its calmative effect to epileptics.

A week passed and Tasya had another seizure, but this time it was different. It was only five to six minutes long, it was not as violent, and the shaking was a little bit milder. We were grasping at straws but both Hillary and I felt that we were finally gaining on her seizures and not losing ground anymore. I also hoped I was not deluding myself.

Hillary's stepfather, Pete, has a great extended family that gets together every year in San Francisco at Christmas time. We were debating whether we were going to drive down there and see everyone and risk being away from the hospital in case Tasya had another convulsion.

What changed our mind was the increasing spread between her seizures and how they were lessening in strength. It was now ten days since her last grand mal so we decided to go for it.

We had gotten a prescription for a suppository form of Valium in case she went into a convulsion on the trip. Hillary packed up for the two day trip and off we went, hopeful that nothing tragic would occur.

The first sixty miles from Tahoe towards the Bay area is beautiful, the road meandering along Interstate 80, going through the rugged, snow capped mountains of the Sierras. We were enjoying the view, talking, singing and having a good time. Tasya and Hillary needed to go to the bathroom so we decided to pull over at a familiar gas station in Auburn, California.

A woman came out of the bathroom less than a minute after Hillary and Tasya had gone in, telling me to get in there quickly. As I rushed there, Tasya was on the floor but strangely not shaking or anything.

"She sat on the floor, started seizing for about thirty seconds, Mark," my wife Hillary, said almost astonished. "But it stopped almost as soon as it started."

"What do we do now?" she asked.

"Let's use the valium and keep her calm while we decide what to do next," is how I responded.

We got the Valium into her and she went into a deep sleep as we pondered our next move. I wanted to turn back and go home. Hillary, ever the adventurous one, said no, we need to go on and Tasya needed it. Our daughter had so looked forward to the trip to see her aunts, uncles, and especially her cousins.

As we got Tasya back into the car, we realized that this seizure was a continuation of the trend of milder and milder "shakes" that were spreading out further and further. We felt deep in our hearts that things were getting better so we decided to go for it and go to the reunion.

It took about two hours before Tasya began to come to but gradually she began to open her eyes and look somewhat coherent. Her first words were, "I'm hungry."

We tried feeding her, but because of the Valium, she had a hard time chewing. She did her best, and after a while, she started perking up and looking clearer. Through it all though, she smiled and laughed at how she felt. Hillary and I both drew on her energy and our spirits rose with hers.

This was the start of a period of recovery for Tasya, one that would last for a few years before the real struggles with her epilepsy would begin. From that moment on, her seizures would only come early in the morning, between 4:00 and 6:00 am everyday. To this day, I wake up around that time even if I'm halfway around the world. To this day, I haven't slept through a night since her seizures started even though the nocturnal seizures are rare.

Still that is nothing compared to what she goes through.

4. NUTRITIONAL PROTOCOLS IN EPILEPSY AND MY FOCUS ON TOXICITY

Our body is a machine for living. It is organized for that, it is its nature. Let life go on in it unhindered and let it defend itself, it will do more than if you paralyze it by encumbering it with remedies.

— Leo Tolstoy

When a lot of remedies are suggested for a disease, that means it can't be cured.

— Anton Chekhov

Probable impossibilities are to be preferred to improbable possibilities.

- Aristotle

There is a great deal of controversy in the epilepsy world about the use of nutritional supplements and herbs for people with seizure activity. This concern is expanded greatly when talking about children. Obviously with my penchant for nutritional medicine, I have my opinions and experience that needs sharing.

Drug therapies are not for everyone, nor are nutritional ones. Tasya likely will not be drug free because of the severity of her seizure disorder but she will likely not need as great of a dose as others nor will she suffer many of the side-effects because nutritional supplements are as much a part of her everyday life as are her meds. The synergy of the two concepts is where I believe medicine, and in particular the treatment of epilepsy, should go.

By simultaneously focusing on potential assaults on her little body by environmental toxicity, I can prevent exacerbations, improve general health, and provide her the best possible platform with which to achieve the highest potential possible in life. Because not all of us are dealt the best poker hands when we start life, many of us and our children still have the ability to achieve a level of greatness if given the opportunity. While drugs try to alleviate negative health issues and resolve problems, it is my firm belief that nutrition and detoxification protocols give children and even adults a boost towards optimal health and ultimately the ability to achieve the greatest potential in our lives.

In today's world, there unfortunately seems to be this barrier between allopathic "conventional medicine" and alternative complimentary health care. Both sides have not only built walls between themselves, they have constructed elaborate moats filled with alligators to prevent any mixing of the styles. This hurts not only the practitioners but the patients as well.

The only way Tasya has been able to progress as far as she has is with the integration of the two disciplines. The proper use of medications (which you will see in the coming chapter was not always the best choice) and biochemically individualized nutritional regimes that have made all the difference in her world. The sad part is I had to do much of the integration, keeping the nutritional part of what we were doing for her away from her conventional neurologist and the medication part away from her alternative docs. This was done to avoid conflict and belittlement from both sides.

In the early days, we had Tasya taking 125 mg of Depakote™ twice daily and then the neurologist had us add 100 mg of Zonegran twice a day as well. While it seemed to help with her grand mals, there was little or no abatement of her nocturnal seizures. Later on in her life, the two drugs seemingly did nothing to stop the drop seizures that were to become part of her everyday life. If anything, they made things worse.

In addition to the meds, as I stated earlier, I started her on taurine. Giving her one gram a day, we did a plasma amino acid test with MetaMetrix Laboratory (see resources) and lo and behold, her levels were at the bottom of the reference range despite giving her such a seemingly high dose.

Many of the studies that I've looked at that show little or no benefits to taurine supplementation are typically low dose models which is most likely why no improvements were seen. They also never seem to address co-factors such as vitamin B6 or C or any other nutrient interactions. Tasya, being the trooper that she is, learned very early on how to swallow capsules. As a matter of fact, she does better than most adults I know.

The other issue I had to address was her generally deficient amino acid levels. I undertook the task of creating an amino acid blend. Amino acids are such a foundational part of health, especially when dealing with neurological disorders; I knew intuitively that I needed to work on this. The first problem I came up with was taste. It was vile and I knew Tasya wasn't going to have any part of it unless it tasted good.

Working with the manufacturer, I came up with a solution using the sweetener sucralose. Now before any of you get up in arms yelling that it's an evil additive, read my opinion paper later on in the book. The doctor who has spread all the rumors about it is selling you a bill of goods and being quite deceptive. Oh, and he is also selling his brand of stevia. Having said that, there will be people sensitive to sucralose, having negative reactions to it. We are all unique individuals but we cannot make blanket statements either positive or negative about something based on anecdotal evidence. What is good for one person may be poison for the other.

The clue that told me I had succeeded was when Tasya dipped her finger into the sample jar of the new aminos, licked her fingers and got ready to dip them in again. The smile on her face told me it was a hit.

Hillary, who had graduated with her second master's degree, this time in counseling psychology, decided that we needed to get this product on the market along with the new line of electrolytes I had developed. Right before Tasya started having her seizures we formed the company, Knowledge Through Solutions (now part of Crayhon Research), to promote new and innovative products that I developed. The amino acid blend was called MyAminoPlex™.

We also regularly had her do what she liked to call her "pee test," a urine organic acid test from MetaMetrix. The results of the first one astonished me and led me on my path of determining whether toxins were at the root of her seizure disorder.

The test came back with a number of abnormal readings but one analyte struck a cord in my brain; it was 2-methylhippurate. This by-product of the detoxification of xylene or toluene (two neurotoxic solvents) was 325% above normal.

How could my kid get exposed to high levels of solvents living in a supposedly pristine environment, and especially since I was so careful about the kind of products we used in our household?

Then it hit me. Two weeks before she had her first seizure, the maintenance workers who were taking care of the condo complex slipped a note under our doors telling us to keep our pets and kids inside as they had sprayed pesticide around the area. A few days after the spraying, Tasya had a 102 degree fever. It was ten days later when the first seizure hit.

Did I stumble upon the answer? Could it be that easy? Well yes and no. I did come across the answer to some other people's seizure disorder but alas and sadly not Tasya's.

Not all was lost though. The path I was going down, while not the perfect answer, did bring many positive results.

In order to detoxify solvents, one of the key components is to use the amino acid glycine in order to bind the chemicals once they are oxidized. The problem that arises is when the toxin is not bound efficiently. I will explain the issue later in the book but the down and dirty truth is that the chemical that is produced by the body oxidizing a chemical like xylene, which is 2-methylbenzoate, is more neurologically toxic than had it been left alone. Glycine combines with the solvent to form 2-methylhippurate which is easily urinated out of the system and is generally safe. It was this marker that was so elevated in my little girl's urine. Since then, US Biotek in Seattle, Washington has developed a simple urine test to look at a wider variety of solvents.

I began a regimen with her that included electrolytes, amino acids, a B-complex, multi-vitamin/mineral complex, as well as taurine and glycine. Improvements started to come shortly thereafter. Her demeanor was better, her seizure activity was lessening, and then came the kicker. Her EEG came back almost normal. Our new pediatric neurologist, was happy. Hillary and I were happy. Of course, Tasya ultimately was the happiest one of all. We thought our nightmare was coming to an end.

Oh boy, were we wrong with that.

Getting back to the issue of toxicity, I had initially thought that Tasya's seizure activity was directly related to the exposure of pesticides she had when she was three and one-half years old. I even lectured about it very convincingly. Alas, I was somewhat mistaken. While the pesticide exposure most certainly did not cause her to develop epilepsy, it may have triggered its onset. What I believe is more likely is that some how, the real reason she developed epilepsy was some sort of toxic interference when Tasya was still in fetal development. There are numerous studies implicating everything from PCBs, mercury, lead, pyrethroid insecticides, and many others to brain abnormalities in developing fetuses.

Can I prove this hypothesis? Absolutely not. Am I off base for looking into it and investigating the possibility? Certainly not. While this may not solve Tasya's problem, maybe it will help one child, one life, somewhere. What my child has gone through, no child should ever have to suffer through. We must use the precautionary principle here (see my chapter on this important policy issue) when defending our kids' futures which ultimately is the future of all of humankind as well as the very planet we live on.

To idly sit back and not discuss or even look into the possibility that my daughter's seizure activity was in some way caused by the environment would be irresponsible given my position in life. To fully lay blame at the feet of polluters and others who deny that toxins could possibly cause her problems would be equally irresponsible. To allow the destroyers of our environment to go unopposed would also be horribly irresponsible.

If my wife and I were to follow the line fed to us by the neurologists that the brain is too complex and you just have to learn to deal with your daughter's epilepsy, we probably would have lost her, as you soon shall see. To investigate and research areas beyond the comfort zone and confront issues potentially uncomfortable for some is the only way my child, or anyone else for that matter, will achieve any sense of victory in the troubling, toxic world we live in.

5. THE YEARS OF FEAR AND DESPAIR

"But what we call our despair is often only the painful eagerness of unended hope."

George Eliot

"At man's core there is a voice that wants him never to give in to fear. But it is true that in general man cannot give in to fear, at the very least he postpones indefinitely the moment when he will have to confront himself with the object of his fear."

Georges Bataille

"Because I remember, I despair. Because I remember, I have the duty to reject despair."

Elie Wiesel

Hillary was now pregnant with our second child. We had wanted a second child for a while, but only when we felt that Tasya was doing well enough that we could give another member of our family the attention they deserved.

Our soon to be oldest daughter was still having nocturnal seizures every week or so, nothing like early on in her life, and nothing too dramatic. Tasya was reading above her grade level and seemed pretty well adjusted for a five and a half year old. Then something changed. Tasya's world was about to change in a way we did not expect and it wasn't good. The next few years were going to test all of us, most of all Tasya.

I cannot recall when she fell down for the first time, but I do remember that we kind of brushed it off as just another clumsy thing Tasya was prone to do. She was a little uncoordinated but we knew that the seizures could not be helping any.

The private school she was in began to call us every once in a while telling us that Tasya had bonked her head or hit her nose into the table. Then we began to see her dropping for no reason, flinging forward, violently at times. We made a panicked call to our new neurologist, asking to see him right away.

He did an EEG on Tasya and it did not look good. The previous summer he commented on how good her brain waves looked but this time she was all over the place, especially when she fell asleep. Her seizure disorder was getting worse.

Early on, when her first neurologist gave her the diagnosis of generalized myoclonic epilepsy, she hesitated in adding the term progressive as it was both unlikely and was probably more discouraging than we would have been able to handle at the time. Now, it looked like our beautiful daughter was on a slippery slope down hill.

It was likely that she would become worse and that her seizures would not be controllable.

Frantic, I began to run whatever tests I could on her, from urine organic acids, to plasma amino acids, blood chemistries and more. I did whatever I could do to uncover why this was happening. Nothing made any sense.

Before the test results got back to me, she had one horrible fall at her school. While walking to music class outside, she had a seizure and went face first into the paved driveway. Hillary and I raced to the school and saw that her face was all bloody, scraped up, her nose was cut and she had an enormous purple knot on her head. We were shocked to say the least.

Our baby girl was going through hell, falling down all the time, and nothing we did was working. Not the nutrient regimen, not upping the meds, nothing

Her drop seizures would come on out of nowhere. She would just suddenly fall or jolt forward. Doing homework was so hard for her as she could not do it at the table for fear of hitting her head or nose.

Then, the drops went away, for a week to ten days at a time. Tasya would be back to her normal self but with subtle differences. She was more uncoordinated, she would trip while walking, and her reading started to suffer.

During this time, I began to get more and more protective of her, stopping her from sitting on high chairs and playing around our yard in places that I thought were dangerous. I was becoming a nervous wreck trying to make sure my baby would not get hurt.

The good times were great though. Then out of the blue, she'd fall down again and get shaky. Her whole body would twitch for hours. Her muscles were firing constantly and she couldn't relax. Bedtime and sleep was the only time her little body would remain calm.

Watching her during the bad days was so hard to do. You just cannot imagine what it's like to see her trying to do something as simple as brushing the hair out of her eyes. Her hands would shake and would rise up to her chest and twitch endlessly.

During the summer of 2002, we went to Orlando, Florida to go to a conference. Seeing that Disney World was there, we took Tasya along hoping she'd get a little bit of happiness. We were lucky that she was having one of her good weeks when we went out there.

John Thoreson a good friend of mine, who works with US Biotek and Pharmax, came to dinner with a bunch of us and sat across from Tasya. Suddenly, her face smashed into the plate in front of her. She began to cry. John's face turned so sad that I remember it like it was yesterday. He told me that he finally understood what she was going through and how Hillary and I were suffering for her. I held my arm across her chest for the next hour as we ate, hoping that I would be strong enough to stop any other seizure from happening.

I decided to let Tasya do the "pee test" again. Another organic acid in urine test from MetaMetrix was ordered. This time the results came back very different than before. Her results showed definite signs of hyperammonemia (elevated ammonia), so we began to work on that with extra arginine (a conditionally essential amino acid).

The striking results showed one thing that I should have noticed from the smell of her urine; her ammonia levels were through the roof. Three markers, citrate, orotate and isocitrate were extremely elevated with citrate being at a level that was at the top of the scale.

Hyperammonemia as it is known, has side-effects that include lethargy, seizures, brain fog, attention deficit, and many other neurological problems. She had all of that and more. A quick call to Tasya's savior, Dr. Richard Lord, elicited the answers I needed to help her get better. He recommended that we try the arginine right away, about 500 mg twice a day. I was at the local Wild Oats health food store a few minutes later. That evening Tasya started taking it. We waited with baited breath, hoping that this would be the answer.

I firmly believe that it was part of the issue with Tasya as one of the potential problems with Depakote was hyperammonemia, that and the amino acids she had been taking. We would never really know, we only had our suspicions.

After about two to three days, she began to improve on the arginine. Her mind seemed clearer and her seizure activity began to lessen. Maybe we did it this time. I also knew that my amino acid formula needed tweaking. I had to abandon the methodology that other amino acid producers used in devising their formulas. I needed to make it better and safer. The next formula, which is the one currently being distributed, has not caused anyone to build up ammonia since. Tasya's experience taught me an important lesson.

This time, I was not going to sit on my hands and wait for something to change with Tasya; I needed to be prepared for anything and everything. I started making calls and the first one would be to my brother Dr. Alexander Schauss, someone who I did not always see eye to eye with. It was time for me to make amends and bring him back to my life as he was also going to be the Godfather to my youngest daughter Anika. I also needed to lessen the stress levels in my life so I could be a better father and husband.

Dr. Dietrich Klinghardt once told me that it was important when dealing with parents and siblings to accept the best of them while forgiving the worst in their personalities and to not judge them for their faults and foibles. None of us are perfect and all of us have flaws. Look at the goodness in people and then and only then will you achieve peace and build back damaged relationships. He told me that at lunch in the summer of 1997. It took me years to understand what he meant. Ok, so I'm a slow learner sometimes.

Alex is one of those types of people who will immerse himself in projects with a passion you don't always see in others. He has gained an international reputation in the field of nutrition, behavior, and health. It was time for the brothers to talk again. Tasya again taught me an important lesson; friends come and go, family is for life.

While discussing things with my brother, I told him that our neurologist mentioned that anything we could do to reduce Tasya's stress level would be helpful. I commented that additionally, I would do anything to help reduce any potential inflammatory or oxidative stress on her as well. He told me about research he was doing on a new product called Acai (pronounced ah-sigh-eee). It came from the Amazon and was a remarkable antioxidant, unlike anything ever discovered in nature. I was willing to try anything for my little girl.

Months had passed since we started the arginine and we re-ran the organic acid test and things finally looked good; unfortunately Tasya was getting worse again.

Tasya was having one of her really bad days when we received a bag of the freeze dried Acai from a friend of Alex. My girl had learned how to take capsules by the handful now and I decided to give it a try. I had her take two capsules of the Acai and waited to see what would happen.

About an hour passed when I went back to check on Tasya and there she was on the floor playing looking like she did on her good days. No twitchiness, no shakes, nothing. She was looking great.

Things began to improve through September, October, and into November. There were some bad days, but they were fewer and further in between. Then it began to worsen again.

My parents came down for Thanksgiving and the second day they were at our house; Tasya began to have her drops again. My mother was so shocked she had a hard time staying in the room. She was in tears. This woman who weathered the bombings of World War II, who lost her father at a young age, learned that her sister was murdered in the Buchenwald concentration camp, and heard that her brother was killed in war was scared to come out of the guest bedroom. My mother, whose own personal health struggles makes her a hero in my book, was overcome with grief. The emotions of seeing her young and beautiful grandchild in the shape she was in was almost too much for her.

By this time Hillary and I were so used to it, we were emotionally numbed. I spent some time with my mother explaining what was going on and how we had to be supportive of Tasya. As the days went on, she saw such an incredible spirit that surrounded Tasya that she came away with the same feeling as we did, that Tasya had an inner strength few people have.

I cannot forget the smile my kid had on her face looking at her grandfather all the while twitching and having spasm after spasm, eyes fluttering because of the seizures but still gleeful that grandpa was playing with her. It still brings tears to my eyes remembering that day.

December rolled around and we were making plans to head back to the Clyde family reunion in San Francisco again but our supplies of Acai were dwindling. Unfortunately at that moment, everyone's supply of Acai was scarce and ours was rapidly dwindling. We gave Tasya smaller doses everyday, trying to make it stretch as much as we could but finally we ran out.

She began to get twitchy again but we were determined to go to the reunion because she so desperately wanted to see all of her cousins, aunts and uncles.

We got to the McCormick and Schmicks restaurant down by the waterfront and waited inside for everyone to get there before we went downstairs to the catering room that was waiting for us. Tasya all of a sudden fell to the ground in front of my father-in-law's sister Dale. This was the first time she saw Tasya have a seizure and it shocked her much the same way it did my mother.

We went downstairs holding on to Tasya as she was going into her twitchy phase. She was slurring and was having problems staying focused on anything. But she so wanted to play with her cousins it hurt. We could not have her sit at the table with them. She had to stay on the floor, protected from falling on her face. It was so hard to watch as her little heart had so wanted to be with her family and be normal. Hillary and I were heartbroken.

Through it all, she kept on fighting, wanting to go to school, wanting to keep being a child. She kept hoping and, more importantly, believing that she would get better. Tasya was right; she would eventually get better but not before things would get a lot worse.

By this time, Tasya was on Depakote and Zonegran along with an array of nutrients. Our neurologist thought that it was becoming more apparent that Depakote was not helping her but rather hurting her as every time we increased the dose her seizures got worse. He put us on a regimen to wean her off the drug and to start the ketogenic diet. I began to research this option and see what we needed to do in order to get her into a ketotic state.

Ketosis is a stage in metabolism that occurs when the liver has been depleted of stored glycogen and switches to a chronic fasting mode during long periods of starvation or when fed high quantities of fat and/or protein. The ketogenic diet is one where carbohydrates are all but eliminated and the person is placed on a very high fat diet. This is the type of diet that was developed by researchers at Johns Hopkins University but is fraught with potential side-effects such as kidney stones, abnormal liver function, high cholesterol, weight loss, dehydration, and bone loss.

Slowly, we began to remove any form of carbohydrate from her diet and to focus solely on proteins and fat. This is also known as an Atkins-like ketogenic diet, one which was showing promise in treating other children as well as adults with severe forms of epilepsy. We were flying alone since we were not getting much help from our neurologist

By mid-February, we finally got her into a ketotic state (confirmed by using urine test strips) but we saw little improvement. She was almost off of Depakote and on the 19th of February we gave her the last capsule per the directions of her neurologist. We waited to see what was next. We didn't have to wait too long.

6. ON THE EDGE OF LIFE AND DEATH

"Lord, make me to know mine end, and the measure of my days, what it is; that I may know how frail I am."

Bible, Psalms 39:4

"People need to be made more aware of the need to work at learning how to live because life is so quick and sometimes it goes away too quickly."

Andy Warhol

"Just as despair can come to one only from other human beings, hope, too, can be given to one only by other human beings."

Elie Wiesel

Tasya went to school that fateful morning of February 20, 2004 even though we knew she was not going to make it through the entire day. Her twitchiness was bad the past few days but she woke up feeling a little better. She so wanted to go to school, to be normal, we had to let her go. It wasn't an hour before the school called and told us she had another drop seizure.

I was at work with Hillary and she volunteered to go pick up our daughter and stay at home with her. My wife dreaded seeing Tasya as she knew how twitchy she would be. Her little muscles felt like they were being zapped by electricity over and over again. By 2:00 pm Hillary called me and begged that I come home right away as our sweetheart was getting worse. Our pediatric neurologist, had us get some Ativan and Valium to help control the shakiness. It wasn't working. Quite the contrary, it was getting worse.

As the sun set, we looked at Tasya with despair. Her shakes and twitches were coming in ever increasing waves, each more powerful than the other. And yet, I can never get the look out of my mind of her smiling at me when I tried to convince her that it would get better.

In reality, I was trying to convince myself despite what I knew to be the truth. I knew Tasya would have to go to the hospital and that something terrible was about to happen.

Finally, at about 8:00 pm she fell asleep so worn out by the constant seizures that even though she was still twitchy, she could not stay awake any longer. Little did we know that she came very close to never waking up again.

Hillary and I went to our bedroom after finally getting our youngest daughter Anika to sleep, which was no small feat. At 10:00 pm we both collapsed, utterly exhausted.

At 11:00 pm we heard that horrible sound coming from Tasya's room. She was going into a full blown grand mal seizure.

While she had these before, having them this early in the evening was quite rare. Usually, the seizure would end within a few minutes. This time, it wouldn't stop.

Twelve minutes into the seizure, Hillary got a hold of the doctor on call who told her to take Tasya to the emergency room right away. My wife dressed quickly as she wanted to get her precious baby to the hospital as fast as she could. I was to stay with Anika as she needed the extra sleep. Kissing Tasya on the forehead I told her that Daddy loved her and that everything would be ok.

I felt like the biggest liar in the world. How could I continue to make believe that she would get better? There was no one out there who agreed with me let alone had any answers.

Agonizing over my complete failure to save my child even though I was going to work everyday helping countless other people, most of whom I would never meet or speak to, get their lives and their health together, I fell asleep.

The doorbell rang at about 4:30 am jarring me from sleep. Rushing downstairs I opened the door to see a Washoe Country Sheriff standing there. I was petrified. Never before in my life have I felt so shocked, so stunned because I believed that he was there to inform me that my angel had passed away.

"Relax, she hasn't died" said the Sheriff instinctively knowing what was going through my mind probably because of the look in my eyes.

"Your phone is off the hook and your wife has been trying to get a hold of you for the past three hours."

I thanked him with what little strength I had in my voice, tears running down my cheeks, and rushed around the house trying to find out which phone had not been hung up. When I finally solved this mystery I phoned Hillary, only to find out that Tasya's seizure was still going on.

There was a sound of true desperation in my wife's voice. She almost begged me to tell her that everything was going to be okay. I knew I had to lie to her again and convince her that yes, Tasya would make it. It tore at my heart.

The doorbell rang again, and there were Pete and Nancy, my in-laws. They were picking me up to go to the emergency room a few miles away. I scooped up Anika, dressed her warmly, and got into the back of their car. Tears of fear and emotion came flowing out. I didn't know how to stop crying.

We got to the emergency room where we were escorted to the bed where Tasya was lying. Her seizure had finally stopped. The attending physician, whose name I ashamedly have forgotten, noted that my little girl's face was red and blotchy and that it strangely looked like an allergic reaction. Calling on her years of training she made the call to give Tasya a shot of Benadryl. It worked.

There is only so far a heart can soar after going through what we had been through that day but we allowed ourselves a brief moment of joy. It was short lived.

Moments later, she began to spasm yet again. "Oh dear God, give my child a break," I begged.

Her face began to have that red and blotchy look again and the doctor tried the Benadryl one more time. Tasya sighed and began to relax. For the moment, she was calm. I wish we could say the same for the rest of us. Almost six hours had elapsed from the start to the end of her seizure. Six of the most excruciating hours anyone should ever have to endure. Hillary stood by her as only a mother could.

Knowing what she went through that night made me ever so proud to have married this woman. I consider myself very lucky.

The ambulance came to transfer my girl to the main hospital from the emergency room near our home. If it were possible to pray any harder, I would have done so. I rode in the back with Tasya, painfully watching the center of my life breathing shallowly next to me while the EMT attended to her. It was not looking good, but he kept assuring me that she was going to be fine. Lying to me was the right thing to do, for at that moment I could not have handled the truth.

We got to the hospital where they escorted Tasya up to the pediatric neurology ER for evaluation and treatment. Waiting outside the ER was one of the hardest things we could have been asked to do. On the wall were postcards from children and their parents who survived car accidents and poisonings, along with an assortment of other emergencies, thanking the staff for all of their help in saving them.

There were also a number of cards on the other wall from parents thanking the nurses and doctors for doing all they could for their child even though they didn't survive. My knees buckled as I sank to the floor wondering on which wall my child's story would hang.

Finally, we were allowed to see Tasya. They had put her into a Phenobarbital coma, hoping that her brain would recover. There was no real answer though to our question of whether she would come out of the coma normal. In reality, they didn't know if she would come out of it alive due to the severity of the grand mal. The attending nurse later told me that she did not expect to see my girl alive when she came back for her next round of duty.

It is another example of lying not always being a bad thing.

After a few long hours, in came our former neurologist, the self proclaimed epileptologist, the one we very much disliked. She was on the phone to the emergency room physician, the one who saved Tasya's life, and was berating her for daring to use Benadryl without her consent.

Slowly, I stood up and walked to the neurologist and told her that if it wasn't for the actions of that doctor, we would be discussing funeral arrangements for Tasya and not discussing what the next few days had in store for her. She quickly apologized to her colleague and asked me what I meant.

After she hung up the phone I explained to her that in all likelihood, it was the Ativan and/or Valium that caused Tasya to go into the grand mal as the more we gave her, the shakier she got. I described her face, the redness and the quick relief Tasya had from the allergy medicine. Surprisingly, she agreed that perhaps my girl was different and may have indeed reacted poorly to the drug.

Furthermore I argued, knowing that once you gain a victory you have to keep pushing, Depakote, the drug she and our current neurologist had recommended for her seizures was not only not helping to control anything, whenever we increased the dosage she got worse. Could it be that the drug could be *causing* the seizures?

"Possible, although unlikely," was all the doctor could mutter. A small victory, but a win for our side nonetheless.

The minutes turned to hours. She lay motionless on the bed. Her breathing was shallow but steady. The monitors kept tabs on her, barely fluctuating. And I continued praying.

The next day, Tasya's eyes opened although you could tell it was a struggle for her to keep them open for even a few seconds. Gradually, she became more alert and finally slurred out words that sounded like "I'm hungry". Words that brought me back to the Clyde family reunion a number of years ago.

The nurses ordered Tasya Jell-O and water as she was not ready for anything solid yet. It would be a while before her body was strong enough to chew.

Drifting in and out of sleep, Tasya regained her strength. It was good to see her beginning to improve. I wish the girl two beds over would have had Tasya's fate.

About half an hour after we had arrived, a young girl about eleven years old was bought in after suffering a devastating seizure while watching television with her family who were visiting relatives in Reno. They had come up from California to be with their cousins. The girl had suffered from a birth defect in her brain that made it unlikely that she would live into her adulthood, something everyone in the family knew, but none were ready to confront.

While Tasya's condition was dire, the other girl was hanging on by a thread. After they stabilized her, they decided that she needed to go back to California to a hospital near the family home as she wasn't going to last very much longer. A helicopter had landed on the roof to take her home. As she was carted out of the room towards the elevator to take her to the top, I thought to myself how apropos that she would be going upstairs as she was likely to meet her maker soon.

My gaze turned to Tasya and I asked her very softly with my eyes welling up with tears, "Please don't leave us yet. I'm not ready to say goodbye."

Just then, the gurney carrying the young girl came back through the doors again. She was slipping away and they didn't think she would survive the trip to the next hospital. It was time for the family to say one last goodbye.

Losing a child is something no parent should ever have to face. The uncle, aunt, mother, father, and cousins of the young girl gathered around her bed, held hands and prayed together sobbing in a tone that can only come of true heartbreak.

When exactly the girl died I was not quite sure, but the empty spot in the ER told me that her life had come to an end. I knew then that I had to redouble my efforts to find a better answer for my girl. There had to be an answer out there.

Tasya finally woke up again and as every seven year old will tell you, staying in bed just isn't any fun regardless of how many cartoons you watch on TV. She wanted to get out of bed and damn it, I was going to help her. I asked the nurse if it was ok to take her on a walk. She smiled and said "go for it" but warned me it was not going to be easy.

I lifted her out of bed and straightened out her legs and had her try to stand up on her own. Her legs resembled the Jell-O she had eaten just a few hours before. I took her out into the hallway where she looked at me defiantly and asked to be placed on the floor where she crawled around much like she did when she was a few months old. She was angry with us, she wanted us to let her be and let her move around the hallway.

Watching her amazed me. Her will to fight on was just incredible. How did she do it despite all that she had been through?

Special? Yeah, she's all that. Inspirational? And then some!

They finally moved her from the ER into the pediatric section where she began to gather up her energy and get stronger and more ornery. The doctor told us that it would be no less than two weeks before she could go back to school as she was going to have to stay on high dose Phenobarbital until we could get her on a new drug regimen which would include starting her on Keppra. I was also convinced we needed to look deeper into nutritional therapies than I had before.

While Tasya was being weaned onto her new drug regimen, her behavior became more agitated and nasty, especially around Hillary. While the seizures dramatically improved, she was changing into someone we did not like. Someone she did not like either.

7. Temper, Temper, Temper

"We boil at different degrees."

Ralph Waldo Emerson

"I have never known anyone worth a damn who wasn't irascible."

Ezra ound

"It was not that she was out of temper, but that the world was not equal to the demands of her fine organism."

George Elliot

Always an energetic child, Tasya was also pretty darned head strong. Hillary and I often debated who gave her that defiant, hard edged streak. My mother swore it was me, Hillary argued it was her genes. Observing Tasya, it was likely to be a mixture of both.

Months had passed since our brush with death and Tasya was slowly getting better. Her drop seizures were still there but not as often as before. Still, whenever we tried upping the dosage on her meds, which now was a combination of Keppra, Phenobarbital, and Zonegran, it got worse. The neurologist agreed that she was indeed a special child and that the meds were something she couldn't handle like other children.

I was too scared to try a strictly nutritional regimen as I saw how fragile she was and I was not willing to risk her life on a whim.

It was at this point he began to work on getting us to come to the realization that there was a chance that Tasya would never, ever really be seizure free or even under moderate control. The fire within my heart was stoked again. I had to find the answer somehow, somewhere.

We always saw a mean streak in our normally happy girl. She could fly off the handle at the drop of a pin; not very often with me, but almost everyday with Hillary.

Sometimes, when going to work, I wouldn't get to the first stop light one mile away from our house before my cell phone would ring. Cringing, I would answer it and I would hear Tasya screaming at the top of her lungs having a full blown temper tantrum.

She not only screamed, she kicked, punched, bit, and threw things at both her mother and her little baby sister. If I came home she would cower in fear as my voice, when used to its fullest extent, even intimidates me.

After she calmed down, we tried to get her to explain why she saw fit to lose it. In all the years we asked, we never got any answer except one. "I just get angry and I don't know why."

One day in the parking lot of Wal-Mart, she was so violent that she caught the attention of an older man who came up to my wife and said that as a psychologist he had seen many children with her type of behavior turn out to be quite psychotic and uncontrollable as teenagers and adults and that we might think about institutionalizing her. Hillary knew, as a counseling psychologist herself that he might be right. I was beginning to have doubts myself. And then the fire inside of me WAS A REMINDER that I had to work harder and be smarter and find some sort of an answer.

Through it all, her drop seizures got less frequent and she seemed to settle into a somewhat normal life, except for the tantrums which became increasingly violent. This worried us as our youngest daughter Anika was beginning to become a target of Tasya's anger.

Time to fast forward to mid-2005. Tasya's seizures were beginning to pick up steam and frequency. The drop seizures were becoming more frequent and the nocturnal seizures were starting to occur again. Were we headed to another crash? We had to find another answer as nothing, not nutritional supplements or drugs, was making any headway. Back to the testing drawing board. Back to the computer to find some answers.

I began to look into infectious disorders, parasites, anything. Lots of leads, especially one into a parasite called *Toxoplasma gondii*. It is the leading cause of epilepsy in many third world countries,[1] and it is carried by none other than the family cat.

The cat. How could I have missed it? Our black cat Thumbsy was Tasya's favorite pet. She was absolutely heartbroken when our kitty died of what the vet described as an apparent brain tumor. Reading up on this particular parasite fit the description of what our cat had gone through at the end of her life. The blindness, her walking around in circles, and all the other symptoms that led us to the vet where her life was ended fit the diagnosis of *Toxoplasma*.

As I read the literature, it fit the bill. Maybe we found the answer after all. That is until we got back the results of the test for the parasite. Negative. Still, because of my research, a man who joined one of the epilepsy news groups I frequented asked if anyone had any ideas about why he might have suddenly developed epilepsy in adulthood. I wrote back asking where he was from and he told us that he lived in India. Immediately I asked if he had heard about this single celled parasite but no response until six months later when I got a personal e-mail thanking me for bringing it to his attention. His doctor tested him for it and when they discovered the marker for *Toxoplasma gondii* they began treatment and his seizures had stopped. Tasya had saved another life by making me research another dead end for her but a life saver for someone else.

Through it all, I was having a problem trying to get the answer for what was going on behaviorally with Tasya. I began to call all of my friends in the field and ask for help. What was I missing and what could I do to help her control her anger? Drugs weren't helping so nutrition HAD to be the answer. How right I was.

8. TODAY AND WHAT THE FUTURE HOLDS

"I don't try to describe the future. I try to prevent it."

Ray Bradbury

"Real generosity towards the future lies in giving all to the present."

Albert Camus

"The present is the ever moving shadow that divides yesterday from tomorrow. In that lies hope."

Frank Lloyd Wright.

Randy Bimsteffer, a gifted and insightful acupuncturist in Denver, Colorado, told me recently that the hardest part of the book would be ending it. Not the writing of an epilogue or writing a final chapter but finding a cut-off point where I would no longer add any additional information about my daughter or the topic of toxicity. He knew me too well. My constant motivation for discovering new truths and by natural consequence, new and deeper questions would make it hard for me to put my pen down.

Mooshy, as I lovingly call her (only when we're alone as she hates it if I embarrass her in front of her friends), is not cured of epilepsy, far from it. She is always at risk for having another drop seizure, or having "the shakes". Her nocturnal seizures, while increasingly rare, still confounds us as there is typically no real rhyme or reason. The uncontrolled temper tantrums which were a daily part of our lives have markedly improved and are now a surprising event and not an expected outcome of her frustration.

We've regained hope for her future compared to February 2004. Things are certainly on the upswing as long as we keep vigilant and continue to teach her how to make the right choices in life which of course is every parent's goal. In Tasya's world though, it is a matter of life and death for her.

While there were times at the beginning of this journey, and certainly in the middle years where we wondered if she would ever lead a normal life, as of today, the future is brighter than ever. My inspiration spent this past summer enjoying those things ten year old girls should be enjoying.

So what has made my wife Hillary and I so optimistic? Partly blind faith, partly observation and partly due to the incredible knowledge base we've gained in the past seven plus years. Knowledge is power. Knowledge sets you free. Knowledge gives you the ability to adapt to a wide array of circumstances and overcome any barriers put in your way.

The goal of the rest of the book is to impart a small snippet of the vast amount of information Tasya has made me learn and accumulate. Our world is fraught with barriers, pitfalls, and bad breaks but knowledge is what will allow each of you to not only help yourself but help others as well.

Looking at her many lab tests, Hair Elements from Doctor's Data, LEAP Food Sensitivity Test from Signet Diagnostics, the Organic Acid in Urine and Environmental Pollutants Panel US Biotek, and the Plasma Amino Acids from MetaMetrix, we began to understand what we needed to do to keep her healthy and raise her seizure threshold.

When we got her Hair Elements test back I was astonished to see an extremely elevated silver level. Looking at the literature (my immediate response to all questions) I found a paper linking high silver to myoclonic epilepsy in an elderly man. Could this be the missing link?

I made two calls, one to Dr. Andy Cutler a Ph.D. chemist and author as well as an expert in heavy metal toxicity and another to Dr. David Quig of Doctor's Data, a remarkably bright and thoughtful person I got to know at a seminar I sponsored called RenoTahoeFest 2004. I asked for their opinion as to what I was seeing and more importantly what to do about it. Both of these brilliant men had insights to share which finally began to make sense of the past six years. First off, we needed to explain the high silver levels in her hair.

After ruling out internal sources like the use of colloidal silver (very dangerous and not recommended by this author) Dr. Quig asked if we had a newer hot tub. "Well, yes we do" I answered. "What does that have to do with anything?" Turns out, many of the newer hot tubs use silver ion generators along with ozone as an antibacterial to disinfect the water.

Dr. Cutler was not sure of this but a came up with a solution to the intellectual dilemma of whether or not it is an external source. The idea was to test my wife and my hair. If we both show up for it then it is likely to be from the hot tub as neither of us exhibits any adverse health issues. If on the other hand neither one of us came up as high, we would need to do a Genova urine metals test (they are the only ones who look for silver in urine) on Tasya to confirm the presence of silver internally. Results of Hillary and my hair elements test also showed elevated silver which told us that the source was our hot tub.

Still, we needed more insight into things. Dr. Quig's concern was focused on Tasya's slightly high cadmium, not the high silver. However, his next question made me understand more about the recurrent problems I was faced with.

"Have you done any tests to determine her glutathione competency? Remember low glutathione is seen quite often with high hair cadmium."

Glutathione, a tri-peptide amino acid is made up of glycine, glutamic acid and cysteine, is a primary detoxifier and antioxidant. If your glutathione is low, then your ability to detoxify toxins or drugs is impaired. Your ability to handle pro-inflammatory oxidative stress, which in turn lowers your seizure threshold, is impaired.

To say that light bulbs were flashing in my head is an understatement. It illuminated the whole road ahead of me and explained many of the issues Tasya has faced over the years.

I looked at her recent urine organic acid test and lo and behold, her pyroglutamate was markedly elevated, a strong indicator that she was not efficiently producing enough glutathione. Things began to fall into place.

Back in March, after an amazing year of improvement, Tasya started having an occasional "shake". She would hit her desk at school with her head or fall to the floor and get that "twitchy feeling" again. Hillary and I were scared that we were going to go through another downward spiral once again.

Were the drugs causing her problems? We asked her neurologist and he suggested increasing the dose of Keppra and despite our counterintuitive suspicion that it was wrong we tried. We were both right and wrong about this.

As expected, the shakes got worse, culminating in a hard fall where she slammed her face into the concrete walkway at school.

Bruised and battered, her face looking like she just got into a boxing match with Mike Tyson, Tasya for the first time looked defeated. She looked at me with tears and told me, "I'm tired of the shakes. I hate having them and I'm scared. "

Our next call to the neurologist was most frustrating and somewhat angering. When asked what to do with her the doctor asked whether we had any Ativan. My wife's shock at this suggestion turned to anger as she reminded him that it was her strong negative reaction to that drug that contributed to her six hour seizure the previous year. When we reviewed medical notes from him, we saw a number of references to this problem so we knew it was something he was aware of.

It was at this low point that my conversations with both Drs. Quig and Cutler happened. I did not need to change her medications; I needed to make them work better. I had the answer to a problem right in front of me.

As I will explain later in the book, the body has a two-phase detoxification procedure. In Phase I, the toxins are oxidized or transformed which creates a secondary byproduct which can be more toxic than had your system left things alone. Your body also has to detoxify the drugs it is taking as well. This prevents the over accumulation of the medications.

In a normal situation Phase II occurs where the new compound (in the case of xylene it would be 2-methylbezoate) is conjugated (bound) to an amino acid like glycine or cysteine (there are a number of others) and made non-toxic and excreted from the body typically via urine (or stool and possibly through the skin) as 2-methylhippurate if the chemical is xylene or toluene. If your system is impaired in glutathione production then over time toxic byproducts of Phase I buildup can occur and BAM, the seizure threshold drops, things spiral downward, and you have this new cycle of degeneration. This of course is an oversimplification of what really goes on as it is a lot more complex than this.

Modern neurologists would not look at it this way and would begin to explore the possibility that the medications need to be increased or changed by trying a new cocktail mixture until control was achieved. The problem with my daughter is that while increasing medications may be the right thing to do for some, she may not be able to handle the increase without negative side effects. What I had to do was increase her glutathione levels so that her body could detoxify the drugs' by-products more efficiently.

My next question to Dr. Quig was "What in your experience is the best way to increase glutathione?" he said quickly and confidently, "whey protein."

It didn't take me long to get over to Wild Oats and pick up some. When I got home I sat Tasya down and told her that whey protein shakes and her were going to be developing a long-term relationship. When she tried the shake, to say she wasn't impressed would be an understatement. She hated it. From there we tried mango smoothies, Jamba Juice, and other concoctions to varying degrees of success. But there were inconsistent problems that we kept coming up with that would be explained later with the results of her LEAP test.

Another quick way to boost glutathione quickly is by taking 500 mg of vitamin C a day. Getting that into her was easy as Tasya has no problem swallowing pills and capsules of medications and nutrients.

Adding that to her pre-existing regime gave us some powerful and immediate positive results.

Within two days the ever-increasing number of shakes and twitches stopped. Her nocturnal seizure activity abated dramatically. Her confidence came back along with an improvement in her outlook, as well as ours.

The first week went by and while we were happy with the results we were cautious as we have had these remission periods in 2003 and 2004 before the seizures returned. Two weeks was the longest time of remission we had back then. Week two passed and there were no shakes. Week three has come and gone and she was still doing better. It stretched to four weeks before a combination of heat (over 100 degrees), hunger, and exhaustion caused her to have another burst of seizures. We boosted her glutathione and were able to gain control again within a day and a half. This was a dramatic improvement over the past few years.

One sure way for Tasya to have a nocturnal seizure or regression test was for her to stay up late and wake up early. That never failed to cause an increase of seizure activity.

Hillary and I went out to comedy club one night and when we got back at 11:30 pm Tasya and Anika were on the couches asleep. The babysitter said that Tasya fell asleep only about half an hour before we arrived home making me pretty sure that I would be waking up that morning to the sound of a seizure.

At 6:30 am I woke up with a start. The sound came from the direction of Tasya's room, or so I thought. I grabbed my robe and raced down the hall to find an empty bed. My first thought was that she had fallen out of bed but when I looked around, I could not find my daughter.

I heard more sounds coming from downstairs and there was my sweetie on the computer playing a game on the Internet.

"Hi Daddy!!!" she said in a bold and clear voice. I asked how she felt and her response was the typical Mooshy response. "Good"

No shakes, no twitchiness, no nocturnal or waking seizures. This despite having a headache the night before which usually was another harbinger of seizures to come. So how did the use of glutathione answer my questions and make me understand why many of her drugs had failed her in the past?

A few practitioners suggested intravenous glutathione to me. Could IV glutathione be an answer here? Yes, if you want to potentially quick fix fraught with nasty side effects. No, if you want real, long-term sustainable results. No, unless you want your child pissed off at you for sticking the needle in her arm every week or more often.

My motto is if you give the body all the tools (nutrients, amino acids and electrolytes) in a biochemically individualized manner by using the proper array of tests you will retrain it to do things right. This can be achieved even if genetics are against you.

Dr. Bruce Ames of the University of California Berkeley, once pronounced that you can suppress the negative genetic expression of a number of diseases through the use of vitamins, minerals, and amino acids. Biochemical individuality used correctly and not being given lip service is the key that I keep getting reminded of everyday with Tasya. This is what allows her to live a normal, happy, and healthy life.

This concept is an attainable goal that takes just a little bit more work and responsibility but is necessary as the current protocol-based medical model is failing. Non-protocol or evidence based medicine is what we need to look for in health care.

Tasya continued to have shakes here and there and they were beginning to get more frequent. Hillary began to dig harder for some answers and came up with a possible explanation for what kind of epilepsy Tasya had since no one else had any idea. Doose Syndrome was one that seemed to fit her more than any other. Once she gave me that ball, I ran with it and searched to find out everything I could about the disease.

Stumbling upon the DooseSyndrome Yahoo group I began to ask questions which surprised a few people in the group as they knew about me from other epilepsy newsgroups out there. My search led me to a name of the doctor who was considered the best in the field, especially when it came to this obscure form of epilepsy.

We decided to take her to Stanford University's Lucille Packard Children's Hospital to see Dr. Donald Olsen, considered one of the best pediatric neurologists in the country. We needed to find out what was causing her seizures and if there was anything else we could do.

The trip was well worth the trouble as we finally felt that we were going to get some real answers. Dr. Olsen, who I recommend heartily, felt that Tasya had a neurocutaneous form of epilepsy somehow tied to her café au lait markings on her shoulder and chest. What this meant is that during embryonic development the skin and the brain fold from the same cells, and at that time something happened to her brain that made her susceptible to having seizures. It also meant that she would likely never outgrow her epilepsy. This was somewhat disheartening to say the least.

It is my deep seated belief that the etiology was caused by something in our environment, something that caused her to develop epilepsy where no genetic component could be found. I am not going to tell you that I am 100% sure of it, but all signs point in that direction. Even if I am wrong, I firmly believe that by working on this book, I may be able to prevent one child and one family from going through what we did.

Dr. Olsen did leave an out though and suggested that we see a dermatologist to get a definitive diagnosis. In his closing comments to us, he felt that she did have all the signs of Doose Syndrome, also known as Myoclonic Astatic Epilepsy or MAE.

He went on to say that looking at her MRI, numerous EEGs, and other tests and observations, he was pretty surprised that Tasya was not learning disabled. This was in my opinion, a testament to the nutritional program we've had her on all these years. His opinion was encouraging to all of us that we were on the right track.

The report following our visit to our pediatrician and neurologist suggested that we change Tasya's drug combination from Keppra, Zonegran and Phenobarbital to Topamax and Lamictal. Dr. Olsen seemed rather surprised that this was not tried on Tasya considering her EEGs. He firmly believed that this combination would be more efficacious than what she was currently on.

We finally decided to have Tasya tested for food sensitivities as well using the LEAP (Lifestyle Eating And Performance) test from Signet Diagnostics. After getting the results back I have to admit an urge to take a stick (stiff and very hard) and whack myself in the head a few times for waiting so long to get the test done.

Children with epilepsy, especially those with difficult to control cases like MAE (myoclonic astatic epilepsy), need to reduce proinflammatory stressors as much as possible. The LEAP Test, available through Crayhon Research is, in my not-so-humble opinion, an important tool to help reduce the effects of foods and food additives on many health issues and in particular seizure disorders.

The synopsis of the LEAP Report that follows is Tasya's. As I have mentioned previously she goes through periods of remission, with little or no seizure or behavioral problems then suddenly begins having temper tantrums as well as atonic and absence seizures for no apparent reason. For years we suspected foods and used an elimination diet with no success. An IgG/IgE test revealed only a minor allergy to egg, a food Tasya has refused to eat for years.

When I found out about the LEAP test I was impressed by the breadth of research done on the efficacy of the test with both Migraine and Irritable Bowel Syndrome (especially those with diarrhea). Immediately I began to look into the value for epilepsy.

The results of the test were both surprising and illuminating. They explained a lot about the triggers that preceded her increased seizure activity and may help to explain some of her behavioral problems.

The foods are ranked according to the test reaction levels with green being non-reactive, yellow being moderately reactive and red being highly reactive. The list of foods being tested includes 127 foods and 23 food additives (chemicals). Some of the reactive foods were expected, some not. Many of the foods that showed high reactivity matched with Tasya's cravings, a classic sign of food sensitivity and allergy.

Here is a brief synopsis of the reactive and moderately reactive foods and additives.

Group	Reactive – Red	Moderately Reactive - Yellow
Vegetables	None	Spinach, Zucchini, String Bean, Eggplant, Pumpkin,
Grains	None	Corn, Wheat
Chemicals	Phenylethylamine	Aspartame, Tyramine, FD&C Red, Potassium Nitrate, Sodium Sulfite, Solanine, Saccharine
Fruits	Olive, Orange	Strawberry, Apricot
Meats & Poultry	Pork	None
Seafood	None	Crab
Flavor Enhancers	Lemon	Mint, Cayenne Pepper
Beans & Legumes	Lentil	Sunflower Seed, Lima Bean, Pinto Bean, Green Pea, Soybean
Dairy	None	Cow's Milk, Blue Cheese, American Cheese
Miscellaneous	None	Tea

Not surprising, over a period of a few days before one increase in defiant behavior, Tasya had consumed crab, string beans, hard cheeses, and chocolates (the latter two being high in phenylethylamine), as well as olives and olive oil, oranges and lemon juice, all of which are either reactive foods or moderately reactive.

We then began to carefully monitor her diet and eliminated all reactive and moderately reactive foods and she seemed to calm down dramatically and became the happy child we always knew her to be. In addition, her seizure activity became almost non existent.

Weeks later, Anika had an ice cream social at her new school and before we could get to Tasya, she had a bowl of lemon sherbet along with a number of red dyed gummy bears and some cow's milk ice cream and soy ice cream. Our expectation was that her seizure activity, especially the nocturnal variety, would crop back up. We were not surprised when that came true that night.

Tasya also began to become "twitchy" with a few absence seizures the following morning. We immediately began to add anti-inflammatory nutrients (Acai, glutathione precursors like glycine and cysteine, and omega 3 fatty acids). In a few hours, she was back to normal feeling relaxed and happy.

We are seeing dramatic improvement in Tasya's life following the ImmunoCalm program that comes with her LEAP Report. The first step was to completely eliminate all the foods with high reactivity. Here is a listing of the common and hidden sources for the foods and additives that were in the Red group in Tasya's test results.

Food	Common and Hidden Sources
Phenylethylamine	Chocolate, red wine, aged cheeses
Olive	Black olives, green olives, olive oil, ethnic foods (Greek, Italian, Middle Eastern)
Orange	Anything orange, orange juice, fruit juice blends, soft drinks, candies
Pork	Anything pork, bacon, hot dogs, sausages, canned baked beans, soups, Chinese soups
Lemon	Baked dessert goods, candies, soft drinks, ice creams, ices, condiments
Lentil	Indian foods, canned soups and stews, veggie burgers.

But it is not enough to eliminate just the most reactive foods; you need to reduce the moderately reactive foods as well. Each LEAP Report includes a complete guide to help find all of the sources of these foods. By eliminating as many proinflammatory reactive foods as possible, healing is more likely and easier to accomplish.

So far so good. Because of the negative reactions she has had when she ate foods that were on the red list, Tasya has become fervent in her avoidance of them. At school, when presented with tempting cakes, ice creams and other treats, she has been adamant in her refusal to indulge. This is what makes us so proud of her.

Between September of 2005 and September of 2006, Tasya has had only five moderate tantrums. This is a far cry from the five to seven she had a week before the test and the subsequent diet. Not only that but her seizure activity is the lowest it has been since her first one in October of 1999. Eight plus years of searching for answers have led us to where we are today.

Tasya walks with a new found confidence, a bounce in her step, and a strong sense of self esteem she has lacked for all of these years. One thing that has not changed is her brave attitude in which she carried a whole family on her shoulders.

Her current regimen consists of:

- 200 mg of Lamictal twice daily
- 100 mg of Topamax twice daily
- 1.5 grams of Taurine twice daily
- 2 capsules of Peltier Ultra Electrolytes twice daily from Crayhon Research
- 2 capsules of MindLinx™ probiotics from Pharmax LLC in the morning
- 2 capsules of the Pharmax kids multivitamin with DHA in the morning
- 500 mg capsule of Glycine
- 1 capsule of Acai Ultra
- 2 capsules of PS Omega Synergy form Crayhon Research in the morning
- 1 300 mg capsule of GlyceroPhosphoCholine (GPC) in the morning also from Crayhon Research
- 1 capsule of Magnesium with CoQ10 from Douglas Labs
- And of course 2 vitamin Gummy Bears twice a day

While this may seem a lot, it really is not when you think of all the strides she has made over the years. There are those in the allopathic world who would cringe at the quantity of nutrients we give our child but these would be the same people who would have us try drugs via trial and error not knowing how they work or whether they would even work at all. As I said before, I am trying to give my child the absolute best opportunity to achieve all she can in this world despite her epilepsy. Anything less would be wholly unacceptable.

The next section of my book deals with toxicity and its implications on human health. It is my firm belief that environmental toxins account for many neurological disorders in children. I know deep in my heart that it is the cause of Tasya's struggles in life and her seizure disorder. The more I know and find out about the subject, the more convinced I am.

By becoming more aware about the subject of environmental toxicity, the better off we will all be, especially our children and their children.

The ability for people to achieve multiple victories in life and for the health care practitioner to win battle after battle for their patients is at your fingertips. The coming chapters will hopefully give you a roadmap to achieving victory over a toxic world.

It has given Tasya and countless others the ability to overcome incredible levels of adversity. Now it's your turn.

PART II

9. THE REALITY OF THE WORLD WE LIVE IN

A HISTORICAL PERSPECTIVE OF TOXICITY

> *"The disadvantage of men not knowing the past is that they do not know the present. History is a hill or high point of vantage, from which alone men see the town in which they live or the age in which they are living."*
>
> G. K. Chesterton

> *"But what experience and history teach is this – that peoples and governments have never learned anything from history, or acted on principles deduced from it."*
>
> Georg Hegel

> *"Who has not fully realized that history is not contained in thick books but lives in our very blood?"*
>
> Carl Jung

The environment is our nurturing blanket that surrounds, feeds and protects us. As Joel Salatin of Polyface Farms in the Shenandoah Valley says "The default in nature is health."[2] That is if we humans do not mess things up by destroying our environment which in turn changes the default from health into illness like I believe it did to my daughter Tasya and to countless millions of children every year.

Lest we think that the destruction of our environment is a recent event, I would like to remind everyone of the age old adage 'if you don't learn from your past mistakes you are destined to repeat it'. If I have learned anything while doing my research for this book is that we are repeating history as though none of it ever happened. Unfortunately, we never seem to learn anything from our past and we are continually destined to repeat the errors of our ways. By learning from our past and seeing what we have done, maybe, just maybe, we can do things differently and avoid the catastrophe that may be headed our way.

We do need to be a little honest as well; our earth is filled with toxins that occur naturally. Volcanoes spew tons of toxic fumes as do forest fires caused by lightning, as well as naturally occurring heavy metals and solvents that are found in our natural environment. These are all things our species has had to deal with over the millennium and to a small degree, we have been able to adapt to it.

It is the man-made, accelerated creation of unnatural toxicity that began when we changed from hunter-gatherers to an agriculturally based species. The change started gradually and is accelerating towards our present mad rush to environmental oblivion.

In the beginning of the agricultural revolution, man used simple tools like the hoe and digging stick. It disturbed the land, but not excessively. We then began to utilize fire to clear out areas of forest to grow more crops to match the increasing demands from a growing population. This was one of the first ways man began to change his environment.[3]

Some may argue that had it not been for this way of living, humankind would not have made the great strides it has over the years. Others claim that the agricultural revolution was the worst thing that happened to our planet. Whichever side you take really does not matter, what does matter is to learn from some of the errors we have made when things have been done wrong.

During the Bronze Age, around 3000 B.C. man began to use wood from the seemingly endless forests to stoke the fires that helped fuel the copper and bronze smelters. Thousand of acres of trees began to be cut down to create the fires needed. With the coming of the Iron Age, it took thirty acres of trees to create one ton of iron.[4] This started to add toxins into the air and water around us, granted not very much compared to today. It was a humble beginning to our pathway of polluting but it continues on to this day.

The Mayans, a great South American civilization, disappeared for unknown reasons but archeologists have suggested that it was due, in part, to their poor agricultural habits of massive deforestation and soil erosion. How much this affected their society is not well known but it does seem to be a contributing factor in their demise.[5]

The next civilization I want to mention is considered by many to have been the greatest one of the ancient world, Rome. While some of the reasons Rome collapsed in the 5th century A.D. were due to a political system that failed and internal pressures, another is the way they decimated their environment.[6] The use of predatory animals for the amusement of their citizens in the Forums caused an increase of rodent populations which in turn lowered agricultural yields.[7] This in turn caused farmers to strain the agricultural system in order to feed the growing empire.

Another issue, more closely tied to the overall discussion of this book is the amount of lead and mercury that the Roman society produced and spilled into the atmosphere. Gold production released large quantities of mercury while silver smelting caused high levels of lead to pour out into the air and water. Strabo, the Roman writer, commented that chimneys needed to be constructed taller and taller in order to force the noxious fumes to be carried further away from the cities.[8] Samples pulled from ice caps in Greenland have shown that lead levels in the atmosphere around the time of Rome's prominence were significantly higher than before or after this period.[9]

Historians have proposed that part of the fall of the Roman Empire was due to the poisoning of their citizens for many generations which caused them to have significantly lower I.Q.s as well as causing a deterioration of the general health of the population.[10] This was also in part due to their use of lead goblets as drinking vessels.

The Middle Ages saw a continuation of this trend of rape and pillage of the forests and the effects of metallurgy on our environment. Georgius Agricola wrote in his book De Re Metallica:[11]

> '...the fields are devastated by mining operations.... The woods and groves are cut down.... Then are exterminated the beasts and the birds.... When the areas are washed, the water which has been used poisons the brooks and streams and either destroys the fish or drives them away.'

Similar events occurred in Holland in the 1580s, Japan in the 1600s, and London as well in the 16th and 17th century. The Thames river was so polluted that trout, bream, flounders and other fish abundant in waters of the 16th century were nonexistent by the 18th century, all killed by the increasing pollution of the next phase of human existence, the Industrial Revolution.

By the 1800s, Britain was so polluted that during the month of December 1879 where smog had encompassed the entire city of London, the mortality rate rose by 220 percent. The city was so blackened by the soot from the thousands of belching chimneys butterflies had evolved to take on a blackened look to avoid predators.[12]

In Pennsylvania, in the Monongahela valley near Pittsburgh, there were an estimated 14,000 smokestacks blowing toxic fumes into the surrounding countryside. The areas around the great steel works were virtually stripped of vegetation due to the pollution. There were no regulations around at the time. No one seemingly cared to control the devastation.[13]

As we moved into the 20th century, many countries began to realize the problems wrought by uncontrolled release of toxins into the environment. Rivers were dying, vast land areas were dead and people were getting sick. Did we stop polluting? No, we regulated it. Instead of releasing toxins in an unregulated manner, the government, ever concerned about its citizens, began to give permission to the companies to dump toxins in the environment but in a more controlled manner.

I may sound jaded, but researching the material for this book has made me so. Luckily, it is not all that bad. We have developed new technologies in many parts of the Western world which help to reduce emissions and protect the environment.

Notice how I mention the western world. What we discovered when the Iron Curtain came down is that we saw the utter devastation caused by unregulated pollution that was the way of the eastern block countries during the Cold War. Vast areas of land had been decimated, waterways like the Vistula were so polluted that it was unsuitable even for industrial use due to the corrosive nature of the waters. In an offshore region of the Baltic Sea, over 100,000 square kilometers were biologically dead.[14]

The litany of damaged rivers, bays, and inlets as well as areas of land destroyed and uninhabitable is almost unimaginable. The accumulation of toxins that started 5,000 years ago is so enormous that it is truly hard to wrap your mind around it. This tragedy, created by our species would be so utterly catastrophic if not for one small detail; the ability of our planet to recover, even from the continuing onslaught of today's industrial monster.

Economic gorillas like China, India and the United States can continue to grow and their citizens can continue to thrive if simple intelligent measures are put into place that allow for our world to heal itself. The reality is that the greater the economic strength of a people, the more effect it has on the environment. This was seen in Rome and now in the industrial powerhouses of today.

Paul Harrison, a noted playwright and director once said: "The poor tread lightest on the earth. The higher our income, the more resources we control and the more havoc we wreck." Rarely have truer words been spoken.

While this brief (and very incomplete) chapter on the history of our toxic legacy is pretty depressing, there are things each of us can do to make the world better and more livable as well as staying hospitable for the numerous generations to come. But before we come to that, we need to better understand the world in which we live in now.

10. TODAY'S TOXIC WORLD

"Unfortunately, our affluent society has also been an effluent society."

Hubert H. Humphrey

"Approximately 80% of our air pollution stems from hydrocarbons released by vegetation, so let's not go overboard in setting and enforcing tough emission standards from man-made sources."

Ronald Reagan.

"We didn't inherit the land from our fathers. We are borrowing it from our children."

Amish Belief

So what is a good definition of toxicity? In the book *Introduction to Toxicology and Food* by Tomris Altug, he defines it as "the capacity of a substance to cause adverse health effects (injury, hazard) on a living organism." He goes on to quote the father of medicine, Paracelsus, as saying "all substances are poisons; there are none which is not a poison. The right dose differentiates a poison and a remedy."[15]

Using these definitions, water and air can be viewed as toxins depending on the amount you take in but when I talk toxins, these are substances that in small amounts can cause serious health consequences. These substances are often times defined by what is called an LD_{50} value. This morbid term is known as the "median lethal dose" of a toxin that will kill 50% of the laboratory animals on which the substance was.

Some toxins like botulinus have an LD_{50} value of .000001 milligrams per kilogram of body weight (making this toxin the deadliest of all) whereas table salt, aka sodium chloride, has an LD_{50} of 4000 milligrams per kilogram. The focus of the book is not on super deadly toxins or on ones like ethyl alcohol which has an LD_{50} of around 14000 mg/kg, but on those in between like arsenic, mercury, benzene, and those whose effects on health are not defined so much by their lethality but by their negative effect on one's health.

While acute forms of toxicity are very important like mercury-laden vaccinations on children, my general focus will be more on chronic exposures, built up over the years, which I find most important. Later on in the book I talk a bit about thimerasol and its possible causative factor in the explosion of autism in the world, but as you shall see in my chapter entitled the Loaded Revolver Theory of Toxicity, I believe that these toxins have been building up in children and that the vaccine may be the straw that broke the camel's back. Not only that but in a later chapter I will touch upon a topic that has become more heavily researched over the years; the idea of transgenerational epigenetic toxicity. This is where a toxic exposure to your great-grand mother may be affecting you today even though no further exposures occurred to any other family members.

I have been on a number of forums on the Internet discussing various issues from politics to immigration, from nutrition to sports, but nothing gets people's rankles up more than the idea of global warming. Rarely do I see a topic more polarizing than this one. Some claim that this is nothing more than a natural occurrence with man having nothing more than a small affect. Others see this as one of the greatest threats mankind will face in the next 100 years. Whichever side you are on, one thing is undeniable; we are polluting our world at a speed that is nothing short of astonishing and global warming may only be a side issue.

As I mentioned earlier, Robert Crayhon has warned me about being so negative and scary, but I have got to tell you that one of the great motivators is fear. And sorry Mr. Roosevelt, your quote, "Let me assert my firm belief that the only thing we have to fear is fear itself," does not hold water here. Our greatest fear should be that in doing nothing we risk all.

Few of us realize the enormity of the situation and the complexity of it as well. Let us look at a few facts:

- According to the United States Environmental Protection Agency in 2002 through their "Toxic Release Inventory" tracking system, over 7.1 billion pounds of 650 different industrial chemicals were released in the air and water, 266 of which are linked to birth defects.
- Worldwide, the estimates approach 80 billion pounds of toxins released annually.
- Some of these toxins affect human health in microgram doses.

Nine individuals not in the chemical industry were tested for 210 different chemicals. One hundred sixty seven of these chemicals were found in at least one of the persons tested with an average number of chemicals found per person coming in at an astounding 91. Most of these chemicals did not exist twenty years ago. This study is known as Body Burden and was one of the first in a disturbing trend of reports defining the scope of human exposure to toxins.[16]

In Body Burden II, also published by the Environmental Working Group (www.ewg.org), the cord blood of ten newborn babies was tested and 287 chemicals were detected, all of which are linked to cancer, developmental problems, and/or nervous system damage.[17] What is most frightening about this number is that the researchers involved believed there were *more* toxins but they were limited to testing to the ones they found. Numerous other reports from around the world have concurred.

These findings should make all of us think about the ramifications for a second. The quantity of toxins in our environment is so great that you can easily, and truthfully, say that every man, woman and child has a measurable amount of toxic chemicals floating around in their blood stream. Many of these chemicals are known carcinogens, have been implicated in neurological disorders, genetic disease triggers, and hormone mimickers, and are causing numerous other health related problems.

Because of this I rarely see the need to test for the existence of a toxin. It is far more important to test for the excretion levels of the toxins. When looking at tests like the U.S. Biotek Environmental Pollutants Biomarker urine test, the worst case scenario is not the person who has markers for solvents (unless they are unduly high) but the person who does not. If they are in your blood, and we must take for granted that they are, *not* having them show up in your urine has to be considered to be a bad thing. In his books, *Amalgam Illness*[18] and *Hair Test Interpretation: Finding Hidden Toxicities*[19], Dr. Andrew Hall Cutler, talks extensively about hair testing and how mercury can look low in a properly run hair elements test (Doctor's Data, Chicago, Illinois) but its presence can cause impaired mineral transport which can mask the true nature of the toxicity.

When we look at the sheer volume of toxins being released each day it absolutely staggers the imagination. It may be hard to wrap one's mind around the numbers but here are a few to leave you thinking.

- An average of 2.3 billion gallons of benzene, a component of many petrochemicals and a known carcinogen, is produced each year in the U.S. alone.[20]
- 56 billion pounds of styrene, another petrochemical which used to make styrofoam, is released into the environment each year in the U.S.[21]
- Over 1.3 billion pounds of one of the most toxic phthalates (a plasticizer) are released into the environment each year in the U.S.[22]
- An estimated 12 million pounds of arsenic and arsenic-related compounds (a toxic heavy metal) were released into the atmosphere in the U.S. in 1999.[23]
- Dentists use 40 metric tons of the extremely toxic heavy metal mercury a year. Because of this use they are the largest source of mercury in our wastewater treatment plants.[24]

As you can see the quantities we release in the United States of just these five toxins are staggering. The worldwide amounts, which are difficult to come by, are even more horrifying.

While pundits will point out that naturally occurring toxic releases from volcanoes and forest fires are extremely high and in many cases higher than man-made toxins, this does not give us the green light to dump more into the environment. Having said that I also do not espouse us going back to Paleolithic times because that is not a realistic option. What we do need to do is to look at our consumption of products that use toxins and begin to reshape our life styles to reflect a more caring and gentler attitude towards our world. In a later chapter, I will give you a series of easy tips to accomplish this goal.

11. THE LOADED REVOLVER THEORY OF TOXICITY

"There never comes a point where a theory can be said to be true. The most that one can claim for any theory is that it has shared the successes of all its rivals and that it has passed at least one test which they have failed."

A.J. Ayer

"Theories that go counter to the facts of human nature are foredoomed."

Edith Hamilton

"Delight at having understood a very abstract and obscure system leads most people to believe in the truth of what it demonstrates."

G. C. Lichtenberg

"Vaccines Laden with Thimerasol Causes Autism"
"Mercury and Aluminum Linked to Alzheimer's Disease."
"Phthalates May Cause DNA Damage to Male Sperm"

These headlines are found all over the alternative health magazines, environmental health journals, in numerous blogs on the internet, and sometimes in mainstream media.

"Perchlorate Levels in the Colorado Deemed Safe by Arizona Governor."
"Industry Claims Phthalates Show No Ill Health Effects."
"No Adverse Health Effects Seen in Industry Funded Research on Bisphenol A."

These headlines are often found in the public media, glossy industry magazines, and on slick corporate websites.

Problem is all of them have some truth in them and all of them are somewhat deceptive. What they truly are, is overly simplistic; sometimes on purpose, sometimes innocently, and sometimes with bad intent.

Our minds are trained in school to easily understand simple one to one relationships. It is easy for us to grasp the concept that sodium causes blood pressure to rise. So the public policy to lower sodium intake was an easy sell. This is one of the reasons that cholesterol lowering to prevent coronary heart disease (CHD) was also easy to gain acceptance even though the relationship is not necessarily true. It's the KISS theory in practice – keep it simple, stupid.

Lest you think this is just about high school dropouts, or uneducated masses, it is not. Many, even in the esteemed halls of higher education, have a hard time overcoming the simplistic, one to one relationship theory. In one of my lectures a few years back, I presented a study, published in a peer reviewed journal, which showed that there was no relationship between elevated iron and coronary heart disease[25] and in the next slide I presented an equally well written, peer reviewed study showing a relationship between the two variables.[26] So what gives?

The two papers were both correct and yet because of the short-sightedness and the inability to escape from the one-to-one relationship model, they both got it wrong. Had they looked deeper and seen that people with high LDL levels and elevated iron were more likely to develop CHD, then both studies would have come to the same conclusion. Conversely, those with low LDL and high iron may have shown no increased risk. The problem with research being published that does not take other variables into account is that public policy gets affected; people act upon those recommendations and may inadvertently adversely affect their health.

In toxicology, the study of toxins, the use of single variable analysis is an old and worn out model that needs to be thrown out the window. This is especially true in the world we live in which is a complex toxic soup loaded with varying quantities of thousands of man-made chemical combinations as well as natural compounds which are being released into the atmosphere. Many of these toxins are detrimental to your health in micrograms (mercury, dioxin, PCB)[27] and some scarily enough, we just do not know what level is safe or not.

We know for a fact that mercury is toxic to humans and animals alike. What we do not really know is whether or not the common chemical phthalic acid (used as a plasticizer in thousands of products) enhances the toxicity of mercury in susceptible individuals. My theory which I have presented at a number of medical conferences is that the answer is very likely yes. We have now added a level of complexity to our equation. No longer are we looking at the simple model of mercury + exposure = adverse health event, but now we have added phthalates so the equation may look like this:

$X*($Mercury + phthalates$)$ + exposure = adverse health event. Wait, where did the X come from? Toxicology is not as simple as to just say that you add the mercury and phthalate exposure together and you get a simple additive adverse health event. In the case of arsenic, adding alcohol to the equation may increase the toxicity by 10 fold which means that $X=10$. In the case of mercury and phthalates the multiplier we use may be 1 or 100, we simply do not know. My gut feeling is that phthalates exert a small but measurable effect of 1.5 on mercury toxicity (there is no published evidence to this assumption, it is just a suspicion). My theory surrounds the interference effect phthalates supposedly have regarding testosterone[28] (which may potentiate mercury's effects) as well as its potential to mimic estrogen (which is protective against mercury) and how this effects mercury excretion.[29]

One of the reasons we do not know what the multiplier is, is because of something we call genetics. Each one of us has a complex code called DNA which helps decide how our cells and our body function. DNA patterns are amino acid chains and the pairings along these chains are called alleles (this is the one penny answer, it is more complex than this).

Let us look at a specific grouping of two alleles called Apolipoprotein E. ApoE as it is called, has been implicated as a risk factor for developing Alzheimer's disease as well as being a marker for an increased risk of developing coronary heart disease. Dr. Boyd Haley has proposed that it is also a marker for the ability to detoxify mercury as well. I would go further and suggest it is a marker for the ability to detoxify a number of other heavy metals and toxins as well.[30]

In this allele pairing there are two amino acid possibilities – Arginine (Arg) or Cysteine (Cys). The nomenclature used to describe this gene pairing system defines ApoE2 as being a pairing of Cysteine with another Cysteine amino acid. ApoE3 is Cysteine paired with Arginine and ApoE4 as being Arginine paired with Arginine. Since we are dealing with two allele pairs this is what the different groupings look like:

ApoE2/2 = Cysteine/Cysteine + Cysteine/Cysteine
ApoE2/3 = Cysteine/Cysteine + Cysteine/Arginine
ApoE3/3 = Cysteine/Arginine + Cysteine/Arginine
ApoE3/4 = Cysteine/Arginine + Arginine/Arginine
ApoE4/4 = Arginine/Arginine + Arginine/Arginine

The theory goes that if you are a ApoE2/2, you are an efficient excretor of mercury and if you are a ApoE4/4 you are a very poor excretor of mercury. In between you have varying degrees of ability to effectively remove mercury from the system.

The majority of the populations are ApoE3/3s which means they are not efficient yet not deficient in mercury detoxification capabilities. This may help to explain why some kids who receive mercury through the vaccinations develop autism. Dr. Haley believes that a great percentage of children with ASD (Autistic Spectrum Disorder) may be ApoE3/3, ApoE3/4 or ApoE4/4, which puts them at a much greater risk of having negative effects from mercury poisoning.

So let us go back to our earlier equation - 1.5*(Mercury) + phthalates + exposure = adverse health event, and we add in say the most common allele pairing ApoE3/3. Since the common theory is that this means that you are just somewhat impaired at detoxifying mercury you would think that the multiplier would be one or maybe at worst 1.5. That would be okay if we were living in a world with low levels of mercury exposure. Since we deem it necessary to dump millions of pounds into our atmosphere annually, I would put the multiplier at 2, with the ApoE4/4 at a multiplier of 4 and ApoE2/2 at a multiplier of .50. So the new equation would look like this 3.5*(mercury) + phthalates + exposure = adverse health event.

Next up are the effects of humidity, temperature, and atmospheric pressure on the toxicity of a compound or element. All of these can have a multiplicative effect that can be many times higher than normal. In some cases high humidity, temperature, and low pressure can increase one compound's toxicity 10 fold and another's may be decreased by half. This field of toxicology is poorly understood because of the way research is done. Laboratory toxicology done on test animals is usually done under very strict control. They make sure that everything is the same in all testing procedures to "keep a level playing field" so that test results can be accurately compared. While this is an important procedure to follow, it can easily miss differences in toxicity amongst many compounds that are important in assessing health consequences.

In one study, laboratory animals were given a toxin and mistakenly the three aforementioned parameters were not being regulated as usual. What the researchers noted was a dramatic change in the LD50 level (lethal dose for 50% of the test subjects).[31] The animals were dying at much lower doses than had been seen in numerous previous studies; some at levels 15 times lower than had been expected.[32] Can you see the ramifications? Industry studies that suggest that their compound is safe may be so in a laboratory under controlled conditions but it can be wildly toxic in the atmospherically uncontrollable world we live in. People in a hot tropical environment may see effects that are lethal while those in cooler climates in the north may see no ill health effects at all or vice versus. The possibilities are staggering.

Back to our little equation 3.5*(mercury) + phthalates + exposure = adverse health event. We will assume that this is an environment that does not increase the toxicity of mercury but adds a little bit to phthalates (1.5). Here is the new toxic load equation - 3.5*(mercury) + 1.5*(phthalates) + exposure = adverse health event (for you math majors I know the equation should be written differently but I'm trying to make this easier to understand).

As you can see, we have added a number of layers to the issue. I talked about the multiplicity of toxic exposure but I simplistically only added two toxins to the equation. In a study published called Body Burden, the average number of chemicals found in their small test group was a staggering 97! As I mentioned previously, we do not know whether the effect of this mix can accentuate the toxicity or not. Unfortunately for us, the evidence that is accumulating suggests that the effect is multiplicative and not just additive. This, in my mind, is the most disturbing thought of all.

Let us say that the accumulation of 97 toxins only has a doubling effect of the overall toxicity of what we are carrying around our bodies. Here is what our toxic effect equation looks like now – 2*(3.5*(mercury) + 1.5*(phthalates) + (other toxins)) + exposure = adverse health event. In this person the toxicity of mercury is 7 times the original estimate and the phthalates are 3 times more toxic.

To put this into perspective let us make some simple assumptions (this is not high science but small estimations). If mercury has a toxic threshold of say 50 and the person was measured with a level of toxicity of 10, standard toxicology would say they were in the "safe zone". Plug the numbers into our toxic effect equation just for the mercury part where mercury now equals 10, we get the following number 2*(3.5(10)) = 70. In this individual, given their genetics and their environmental situation we now are above the safe zone of 50. We now are primed to have an adverse health effect.

There is another concept we need to add into the mix that makes this even more complex and that is the concept of chance. Chance is the curve ball we need to throw into our toxic effect equation. In the world of science there are a number of unknown effects out there. As advanced as our understanding of the universe is, we are still babes in the woods.

Say we have two individuals who have the identical score of 70 on our equation. One person develops cancer; the other has a mild case of chronic fatigue. Since we figured in genetics, environment, and toxic load, why would their expression of disease be so vastly different? This is where chance comes into play.

Chance does not necessarily mean some outside force we cannot see, feel, or hear. It could be something as simple as having a particular meal at the right time, or the wrong meal at the wrong time. How many times have you been in your car and saw someone go through a red light in front of you, narrowly missing your car? Had you been there one second earlier, bang, an accident. Some may call it serendipitous, others fate, others still may say it is luck. Who knows?

Using our final equation person #1 is lucky and their final multiplier is .9 because they just happened to have started a diet that, without them knowing it, helps them to detoxify mercury. Their final number of the toxicity of mercury is 70*.9 or 63. Toxic, but just over the top.

Person #2 is not so lucky. They just had a tragedy in their family (grandmother passed away) and they just got a new boss at work who is a rather unpleasant sort of person. Their stress level just went up and their final multiplier is 1.5. Not a big jump but it does make a difference as you shall see. Their final number of the toxicity of mercury is 70*1.5 or 105, double the safe load. Person #1 develops mild fatigue, person #2 develops cancer.

So, how do you understand this theory within the greater scheme of things? How can a health care practitioner explain this to their patients? My goal is to give you a simple visual concept that hopes to answer this complex issue.

When the industry says "there is no evidence that the use of our product has any adverse health effects" or when the vaccine manufacturers claim that "the use of thimerasol had no link to the increase of autism" they are somewhat correct. But what about the patients who swear that their kids regressed horribly after the inoculations? They saw a real event. It really happened. They are telling the truth but science is skeptical because they cannot create a toxic equation that can relate to the event. So what are we seeing here?

This is what I like to call the "Loaded Revolver Theory of Toxicity".

Think for a moment that each exposure to toxins begins to fill the chambers of a revolver with loaded bullets ready to be fired if the trigger is pulled when a bullet is in the right (or wrong, depending on how you look at it) chamber. Chance keeps rotating the chambers, kind of like a twisted game of Russian roulette. Each time we get exposed to a toxin, we either load another chamber with a bullet, or we increase the power of one of the bullets already there.

When we use cosmetics laden with phthalates, or live near a capped waste dump loaded with methylmercury, or drink water laced with diazanon, we add to our loads and fill the chambers of our toxic revolver. You can load a gun, but unless you pull the trigger, little or nothing happens.

So what pulls the trigger on our toxic revolver? "Trigger pullers" vary from stress to vaccines, infection to diet, an accident or another toxin to an unresolved emotional event from the past cropping up. The catalysts, as they can also be called, do not necessarily have to be a single event like a vaccine, they can be a long slow pull of the trigger like a poor diet. Slowly apply pressure to the trigger or give it a quick pull, same effect, different time frame.

Sometimes only one chamber has to be full to get an adverse health effect. This is where chance comes into play. Unluckily, one person may be trying to live the non-toxic life and they do their best to eat right, exercise, and avoid bad things yet they get sick. The revolver just happens to be loaded when the trigger is pulled. Other times the person gets lucky and they can get away with five loaded chambers, but one empty one and that is the chamber that keeps coming up when the trigger is pulled. If we have every chamber loaded, luck is not the lady tonight. You get sick and often times with devastating consequences.

The problem I see today is that we are loading our toxic revolvers at an alarming rate. We also cannot kid ourselves and think this hasn't been happening for as long as we have been upright and walking. The Romans drank from lead goblets, burned fires indoors, and ate foods that were toxic or filled with bacteria, parasites, and viruses. The Industrial Revolution is over 300 years old and the pollution that filled the air in London in the later part of the 18th century was worse than it is today. Volcanoes and forest fires add their natural toxicity to the mix all the time as well.[33]

Still, today's mix of newly formed chemicals, billions of combustion engines spewing toxins into the air, our laziness in using pesticides, insecticides and fungicides where they are not needed, and the vane and ignorant use of toxic perfumes, cosmetics, antiperspirants and the like, has made our world the most toxic ever. Especially since volcanoes, forest fires, and other natural toxin pumps have not gone away either.

When children are born, their chambers are supposedly empty, or at least not loaded with particularly powerful bullets. Some may have the ApoE4/4 gene making them more susceptible to mercury toxicity from vaccines, loading a chamber or two. In today's world, when the mother ingests poisoned fish, laden with mercury, PCBs and other toxins, she begins to load the revolver. Add her cosmetics with phthalates that can affect the development of the fetus and we begin to see how our children are being given an unfair disadvantage in that they start life with almost a full gun, ready to fire at anytime and strap them with a disease like autism, ADHD, asthma, diabetes, and other disorders such as obesity.

Recent research has added another blow to our specie's health. Scientists have discovered that the effects of the toxins can be passed on from generation to generation, not related to DNA damage but the way I look at things, loading the revolver of children whose parents have not even been born yet. So while we are seeing increases in a number of childhood diseases like asthma, diabetes, and autism due in part to toxicity, what have we done to our grandchildren and their kids?

My parent's contemporaries were called, "The Greatest Generation" for their sacrifices in World War II. I lament that my contemporaries whose drive towards convenience and utter disrespect for their environment will go down in history as "The Worst Generation" for the legacy we are leaving our children and grandchildren.

It is our duty to stop the madness and deny future historians with this depiction of our lives. Section three of this book is meant to show you how to accomplish this in your own life as well as how you absolutely, positively can make a global difference one person at a time. There is a lot of hope out there but time is quickly running out and the biggest revolver of all is pointing straight at humankind and the chambers are filling rapidly.

12. Aging and Toxicity

"You can only perceive real beauty in a person as they get older."

Anouk Aimée

"When you are younger you get blamed for crimes you never committed and when you're older you begin to get credit for virtues you never possessed. It evens itself out."

J. F. Stone

"The older you get the stronger the wind gets — and it's always in your face."

Jack Nicklaus

With the aging of the industrialized world's population, a lot of focus has been pointed at doing something called compression of morbidity, which is to push all the diseases of aging to as small as possible period at the end of life. Much of what is going on, according to Tom Kirkwood in a BBC lecture, is that we are trying to increase our "health span" while leaving the life span intact and as is. The real problem with this approach is that we are trying to uncouple health and aging. They are really one and the same. Let me explain

What is aging really? It is the accumulation of how many "hits" our cells take from the numerous toxins it encounters from radiation to solvents, from heavy metals to stress and infections. Author Nick Lane in his masterful work "*Oxygen, The Molecule that made the World*" gives a beautiful example of aging.[34] Say your cells can withstand 100 of these hits before dying; doubling the toxicity (his case uses radiation) halves the life of the cell. He then brilliantly puts aging in a whole different picture. Take time to soak in the following paragraph, it is absolutely brilliant.

"Our biological age equates to the number of 'hits' we have taken. This is turn depends on how we handle oxygen, or, more particularly, oxidative stress. In other words, old age is not a function of time, but a function of oxidative stress, which tends to rise over time. Thus, we ought to be able to prevent degenerative disease if we can prevent oxidative stress. To find a cure for dementia, we should forget about the genes that increase our susceptibility to dementia, and look instead for genes – or other factors – that can protect us against oxidative stress. In so doing, we stand not only to prevent dementia, but at the same time to ward off other age-related disease such as cancer and diabetes."

Aging is not a function of time. What a profound statement. It is basically the accumulation of all the errors of our ways. Some of these errors are our fault (smoking, drinking, poor diets, and microwaving plastics to name a few) and some we are not in control of as individuals (environmental pollution, poor soil nutrient levels, solar radiation). None the less they are faults that our cells encounter constantly that we have to deal with. Reducing toxic exposure is a first step, flushing them out of our bodies is a second step, and increasing our ability to handle oxidative/toxic stress in the future is a third step and the most difficult of all unless we follow the rules of biochemical individuality which I make mention of often in this book.

When I acknowledge that we have to remove the load of toxins in our body, two sayings that my late mentor, John Kitkoski always used to exclaim come to mind:

You can't carry two tons of manure in a one ton truck
and
You can't run a Cadillac on a Volkswagen diet

The first saying is an obvious one. You cannot carry a load of toxins that the body was not designed to handle. The second one means that your bodies are high performance machines that cannot be fed crap and then be expected to run smoothly. If your car needs premium gas and you give it regular, you are going to prematurely age its engine and you won't get the energy output you expect from it.

What astounds me is how relatively bright scientists, doctors and nutritionists make comments like "you can get all the nutrients you need from your diet and the RDA (recommended daily allowance) is all you need for healthy life." And they can do this with a straight face. It could be one of the most dumfounding statements imaginable considering the research and knowledge we have.

One of my favorite shows on television today is one called "Myth Busters" on the Discovery channel. In it two guys have fun destroying common urban legends by testing the myths and seeing if they really are true or not. Without going into great detail I want to arm the reader with a couple of facts that will allow you to win an argument with anyone that tries that line of thought with you in the future.

Myth #1 – The Recommended Daily Allowance for nutritional supplements is "*the*" guideline to follow to determine what you need everyday. A few problems with that thought come to mind. The RDAs are supposedly based on normal people. Normal in what sense is my first thought. The so-called "normal" person that needs the RDA and nothing more is a person of average build, height and weight (for males 5'8" about 150 lbs – females about 5'3" and about 115) with no bad habits (smoking or drinking), who exercises moderately, has no stress and lives in a healthy environment. Some of you probably have already spotted a few errors in their ways.

First off, how many average people are out there? Secondly, you better be living clean and not do anything wrong, ever. Remember you are the accumulation of all your past mistakes. Third and here is where they screwed up the whole argument – NO STRESS AND A HEALTHY ENVIRONMENT!!! Excuse me? Where the heck are you going to find someone like that? I can guarantee you that this person does not exist.

At one of my lectures in 2005, I asked the audience which was filled with health care practitioners from around the world, how many of them regularly saw 5'8" 150 pound men, with healthy diets, good sleeping habits and little stress? I swear you could hear crickets chirping in the lecture hall (just before everyone busted out laughing).

Hold on Mark, I know people who are relatively stress free and live in a pretty pristine area you might remark. Hogwash I say. Negative stress or positive stress is part of all of our lives whether we like it or not. Filing your tax return is stressful, going to the store and trying to find a parking space or watching television (this could be the worst) are all stressful. Sorry but that argument does not hold water. Stress is an everyday issue that most everyone faces.

As for the living in a pristine environment, sorry but that is impossible in today's world. The March 2005 cover of Discover magazine should have put a total kibosh on that notion. It shows how pollutants can travel across the Pacific Ocean from China to the west coast of the United States. About five or so years ago, when I lived in Lake Tahoe one of the supposedly most pristine places in the U.S., the sands of the Gobi Desert from China fell from the sky! They had traveled thousands of miles over the Pacific to visit us and choke our skies.

Want more proof? Did you know, that the land mammal with some of the highest concentrations of mercury is the polar bear? That might be explained if by chance they lived near a coal burning plant or maybe their dentists filled their cavities with amalgams made with mercury. Many believe it is because of the fish diet they eat. That could well be but my suggestion to you is that it isn't the whole answer. Mercury can travel around the world in the atmosphere for up to two years and where it falls, nobody knows but a theory is that certain conditions like the extreme cold of the Arctic increases the drop out rate.

Toxins can and will increase the needs of many nutrients not just because of the increased demand of detoxification pathways but because some of these toxins can block enzyme pathways and other metabolic functions causing an increase in needs for many nutrients.

Myth #2 – You can get these nutrients from your diet. Maybe 50 years ago, but certainly not today. There is ample evidence that foods that are readily available in our grocery stores are not as nutritiously packed with vitamins and minerals as they were in the 1950s. Anyone remember what a ripe orange tastes like? What we see in our stores today is a gassed orange that was picked green. Lots of vitamin C? Maybe and maybe not. There is a large variance in the quantity of vitamin C in many fruits and vegetables so what you think you are getting is not necessarily what is really there.

Of course, there have been numerous studies showing that organically grown foods are somewhat higher in nutrient content than their conventionally grown counterparts. Add the fact that they do not use dangerous pesticides and you get two good reasons for choosing organic.

Myth #3 – All you need to do to stem the tide of aging is to load up on lots of antioxidants because oxidation and the production of free-radicals are the cause of aging. Boy, wouldn't that be nice, but alas, it is not that simple. As a matter of fact, in this case, too much of a good thing is dangerous. I have seen countless train wrecks of people who have done high dose IVs of glutathione who have crashed afterwards and took years to recover. Taking lots of antioxidants can cause more oxidative stress!

Wait, you are doing it again Mark, making my head spin with what seems like an oxymoron. Antioxidants causing more oxidation makes no sense and you are right it does not at face value but that is exactly what can happen. Here is how that works:

Metallothionine and heme are made through a signal that is produced by the oxidation of thiols. This occurs when the levels of antioxidants fall low enough and oxidative stress increases. An example of a thiol-regenerating antioxidant is N-acetylcysteine (NAC).[35] If the thiols are not oxidized then you lower the body's natural response mechanisms because the floating antioxidants should be thought of more as a scattered mob than an evolutionarily guided machine. Our bodies have developed countless protective mechanisms over the millennium to protect against oxidative stress. We would be foolish to think that by just adding high dose antioxidants we could better our natural defenses.

Another issue why the over use of antioxidants may cause an acceleration of aging is in people with heme oxygenase deficiencies. (Heme oxygenase is an enzyme that helps the body dispose of heme and protects organs, especially the lungs, from the effects of oxygen).

In these individuals, the dampening of this response may increase inflammation causing more damage to the system. How many of us have an impaired heme oxygenase pathway is unknown but it is commonly agreed that as we age this becomes less active so in the elderly excessive antioxidant use may be harmful.

Before you all get up in arms, note how I used the word "excessive" and not normal or rational antioxidant use. I also do not espouse the theory of blanket supplement recommendations because of that quirky little theory of biochemical individuality. Before throwing the kitchen sink at something, determine if you are working in the kitchen or not. Lab testing to find out what you really need is more intelligent.

Instead of just rushing out to buy tons of antioxidants, the better solution is avoidance of those things that create oxidative stress like toxicity. Another way to improve our longevity and reduce free-radical damage is to improve our detoxification pathways. I will cover those techniques in the next section of the book.

13. Transgenerational Epigenetic Effects of Toxicity

Is our species doomed?

> *"Children's talent to endure stems from their ignorance of alternatives."*
>
> *Maya Angelou*

> *"What is a neglected child? He is a child not planned for, not wanted. Neglect begins, therefore, before he is born."*
>
> *Pearl S. Buck*

> *"Once you bring life into the world, you must protect it. We must protect it by changing the world."*
>
> *Elie Wiesel*

The horror writer Stephen King has written a number of books and short stories about the end of our stay on earth but I do not think his fictional work can hold a candle to the potential reality of what we have done to our world with our incessant dumping of toxic waste into our environment. What science has begun to discover about what we have done to our world has absolutely staggering consequences.

In a study published in the highly esteemed journal, *Science*, researchers led by Matthew Anway found that fetal exposure to certain endocrine disrupting toxins not only affected the individuals exposed in the womb but in subsequent generations.[36]

The fourth generation of rats tested had the same damage as the exposed rat in the first generation with no additional exposure to the toxin. The inheritance of the damage was not to the DNA but by altering patterns of DNA methylation. DNA methylation is a chemical process that changes the way the DNA works without changing the genes directly. This process is inheritable which makes it so important to research.

This transgenerational epigenetic effect (which is the process that allows one to inherit a trait without changing genes themselves) makes detoxification of individuals, especially those of child bearing age, more important than ever. DNA methylation is one type of transgenerational epigenetic effect.

Now let us ponder what the previous paragraphs tell us. Not only are we creating health problems for us today, we are cursing not just our children, but our great-great-grandchildren. We cannot even begin to fathom what our toxic world means to future generations.

To repeat myself: My parents were called the greatest generation; our generation may be called the worst. The legacy we are leaving is not a good one. The even scarier proposition is that, the way we are going, there may be no legacy left.

To fully understand what we mean by transgenerational epigenetics we will have to define the noun epigenetics and the verb epigenesis.

Epigenetics is basically the study of the formation of a new event/germ/cell/life form/genetic expression not seen before, it is the study of heritable changes in gene function that occur without a change in the sequence of the DNA.[37] Epigenesis is how it started and what made this event occur.

Here is a simple example:

Say we have a person exposed to chemical A. It causes his DNA to reduce the number of, quality of, and mobility of his sperm. This is considered an epigenetic effect. It would not have happened unless chemical A was somehow absorbed into the body and allowed to enter the person's cell where the DNA resides.

A transgenerational effect is where this initial exposure continues influencing his offspring to have the same sperm damage without any additional exposure to chemical A.

We are exposed to thousands of chemicals everyday, many of us walking around with two to three hundred floating through our blood stream, not knowing what effects it is having on our health much less the expression of our genes. They are an experiment gone crazy.

Lest we think that this is a just a recent event, think about the output of toxins from centuries gone by as I mentioned in my previous chapter on the history of toxicity. The Industrial Revolution went on for centuries dumping toxins unregulated. Our great-grand parents are still with us in ways we may not really want.

The effects of any one of these chemicals can be devastating. What we are learning in the field of toxicology is that the combinations of chemicals coursing through our veins may be even more devastating to not only our health today, but to the health of generations to come.

To paraphrase the great psychologist B.F. Skinner; "We are products of our environment." He needed to add that our environments are certainly products of us. Hopefully, the product of our environment is not as bad as it looks like it will be.

14. A MORNING IN THE LIFE OF TWO TOXIC COUPLES

"The best friend is likely to acquire the best wife, because a good marriage is based on the talent for friendship."

Friedrich Nietzsche

"There are more truths in twenty-four hours of a man's life than in all the philosophies."

Raoul Vaneigem

"Our growing softness, our increasing lack of physical fitness, is a menace to our security."

John F. Kennedy

One of the most common comments I get while doing consultations with doctors and their patients is, "I'm not around toxins so how did my test results reveal so much of that stuff in my body"? It just does not make sense. Some claim to eat organic, are careful to avoid bad foods, drink bottled water (that's a joke I'll talk about later) and they do not use bad chemicals.

So what gives?

There is no place left on our planet where environmental toxins have not touched. When you realize that polar bears are being found with high concentrations of mercury as well as Inuit women of child-bearing age in the Polar Regions of our planet,[38] you begin to understand the scope of the dilemma we face. It gets worse my friend, much worse as you dig deeper into our everyday lives and habits.

I spent weeks debating how I was going to present the information but nothing seemed adequate. Do I lay it out like I do in my lectures? Maybe I can do an impersonation of Jack Webb in one of my childhood favorite TV shows, *Dragnet,* and just present the facts ma'am. If I did that I'd break the Crayhon rule of not boring you.

Ranting and raving certainly would be exciting and if I throw in some controversial information I could make heads spin. The problem with that idea is you might get turned off by that style and the real purpose of the book is to open your minds up to what is really happening around you, not to close your mind because of my opinions.

As is my habit, the shower is where my great thoughts come from. One morning I looked at my bottle of shampoo and conditioner and said to myself, "Mark, most people don't realize that by using the wrong shampoo, they are starting their day with a toxic exposure." Excitement came over me as I realized I had a way to explain to each of you how many exposures you get each day. I needed to trace a morning in the life of an everyday couple, a male and a female (you women are in for a shock).

Another issue came up in my mind because I cannot just be the doom and gloomer again. I needed to show you how not get caught up in the toxic steam bath our everyday lives have become. The second couple will trace their morning while avoiding as many of the toxins as they could. What you should come away from in this chapter is how easy it really is once you get into the swing of things.

Here we go!!!

Patty and Donny are a moderately happily married couple in their 30s who try to live a reasonably healthy life. They do not smoke, only drink a glass of red wine once in a while (hey the studies all say that it's good for you don't they?), they exercise every day, and they eat what they think is a well balanced diet. They have a few health issues such as those twenty pounds of weight they just cannot seem to get rid of and aches and pains that the numerous meds they are on do not seem to be covering up anymore.

Oh, yeah they have a hard time waking up in the morning, having to hit the snooze button two or three times and let us not get into the problems they both have getting to sleep at night. Come to think of it they both feel a little less energetic as they did when they were in their 20s which was not that long ago. Sex, yeah, we remember that. It is not that we do not want to; "we're just too tired to be intimate anymore" is their excuse.

Donny wakes up first, although not without a struggle. It is 6:00 am and he has to get out of the house by 6:45 so he can get on the highway and drive an hour to be at work by 7:45 at the latest. He does not really have to be at work that early but darn it, Donny wants to move up in the corporate world and not get left behind so he makes sure he is the first one in.

Before he even goes into the shower, he absolutely, positively must have that first cup of coffee. Without it, he gets a headache; he feels grumpy and worn out all day long. He also takes his meds, one statin to control his cholesterol which at 180 mg/dL isn't high but his doctor just heard a lecture from a top pharmaceutical company's rep that claims real benefits for men in their 30s (even though the data is pretty skimpy), and the other is a time-released prescription for something he does not remember he had. The time-released medication uses phthalates in its coating so he'll be adding that plasticizer to his intestinal tract. He pours the tap water into the Mr. Coffee machine to start the brewing process. Here are exposures #1, 2, 3, and 4 for poor Donny.

The water contains diazanon (a pesticide) and perchlorates from jet fuel. More about that when Patty gets her cup of joe.

The coffee, which they ground a few weeks ago, has gone somewhat rancid because they did not store it in an air tight container so the oils from the beans are dried and oxidized. To top it all off, the coffee maker has not been cleaned in a while and bacteria are growing inside which makes its way to the coffee. So Donny has added four toxic exposures to his day already. Bacteria, pesticides, jet fuel additives and rancid oils.

Donny has his cup of hot java and heads to the shower. He gets into the shower, turning the water as hot as he can stand it, gets his hair wet and opens up the shampoo bottle to wash his hair. He loves the smell of the Granny Smith apples from the shampoo and he feels as totally relaxed as he will any other time of the day. Unfortunately, Donny has just added two more toxic exposures to his day with the shampoo that contains phthalates along with other solvent toxins and with the hot water that is vaporizing the chlorine which he inhales deeply into his lungs. Nine toxic exposures and Donny has only been awake for one-half hour.

As he looks out the shower doors he sees Patty going off to her three mile run as she does everyday. Since it is raining Patty puts on her Gore-Tex™ jacket. Her run is the same as everyday, down the street to the main arterial of her town, Main Street. The traffic is heavy but the streets are nice and level as opposed to the hills on the less congested back roads. Of course, she never runs on the sidewalk as the cement is harder than the asphalt the cars drive on (it really does not make a difference). It feels good to get out and Patty feels more relaxed than she will at any other time of her day, and isn't that why people run? Poor Patty, she just exposed herself to a number of toxins on her run.

First off, her jacket is made with peroflurocarbons (PFCs) which have been linked to elevations of cholesterol and heart disease.[39] Secondly, she inhaled a couple of toxins from the fumes of the diesel trucks and cars including benzene, styrene, toluene and fine particulates which have been linked to an increased level of asthma in the world's industrialized countries. Patty's healthy jaunt around the neighborhood has encumbered her with six different toxic chemicals in the half hour she has been awake.

Donny hops out of the shower and puts on some deodorant which has that manly musk smell (phthalates and other solvents), he puts some jell in his hair (more phthalates and solvents) and he shaves with shaving cream also laden with that familiar plasticizer.

Three more exposures which bring us to twelve and again he only just started his day.

Back home, Patty and Donny normally would have had breakfast together, but darn it, life is hectic and Donny has to get to the office early to finish the report the VP of marketing wants today. It is ok, Burger King is around the corner and he can pick up an egg sandwich and a cup of coffee. The oil at the local BK has not been changed today even though it is supposed to have been, so the potato nuggets are coated with rancid oils and partially hydrogenated fats. The fat content of the meal is about 50% of the recommended daily allowance in one meal. Oh and the coffee uses the same water he used earlier to make his cup. Add four more toxins to Donny, sixteen and counting.

Patty is about to catch up to her husband with her exposure in a big way. First the shower which like Donny's, adds three toxins to the mix. She runs her own small accounting business and is meeting with some potential new clients today so she needs to look good. Out comes her array of cosmetics, hair sprays, and perfume. Ah, the sweet smell of her $100 bottle of French perfume. She just loves the aroma and it makes her feel like a queen. It also is packed with phthalates, solvents and oh yeah, the cosmetics have small amounts of hormones as well.[40]

Don't get me started on the toxic stream emitter aka, hair spray. Just inject the stuff into your veins instead of inhaling it and polluting the lungs. Feel the wheeze!!!

So where is Patty on the toxic chart? Thirteen and counting and she has not had that yummy breakfast which is awaiting her in the kitchen.

Unlike Donny, Pat makes sure she has breakfast every day as her European born parents stressed breakfast to her. She used to be a caffeine junky but now it is decaf for her. Oops, it has been decaffeinated using acetone, yummy. Also, she gets her water from the kitchen faucet with its traces of perchlorate which the governor of the state she lives in (Arizona), Janet Napolitano, said that it "poses no threat to the public".[41] How reassuring but how wrong she is. Research has suggested that perchlorate concentrations greater than one part per billion (ppb) in drinking water pose risks to human health, according to EPA's draft toxicological report issued January 16, 2002.[42] I can honestly tell you that perchlorate levels in the waters coming into Arizona are definitely higher that 1 part per billion. In fact, their guidelines have an acceptable level of fourteen parts per billion! That is fourteen times what the EPA says is healthy. Shame on Arizona's governor for misleading her constituents.

So we see Patty is up to fifteen toxic exposures by the time she gets out the door to go to work.

Let us look at our other couple, Bernice and Stan. Both are also in their 30s but they feel pretty darn good about their health because they try to avoid as many toxins as they can without being paranoid about it. Less stress is always a good thing in their household.

Both of them wake up at 6:00 am and bounce out of bed after a great night's sleep. Bernice and Stan also like a cup of coffee to start their morning so they head to the kitchen and brew some freshly ground coffee by pulling out the beans from the air-tight container in their fridge. This keeps the beans and the oils fresher and avoids the rancidity you get from leaving coffee grinds exposed to air. The water they use comes from the faucet but they have a reverse osmosis water purifier which removes many of the toxic chemicals normally found in their neighbor Patty and Donny's house. No big toxic exposures yet.

Both of them hop into some sweats and go out the door for their morning run. They wave at Patty who jaunts off to run on Main Street. Bernice and Stan go one block over on a hilly side street with a few pot holes but only a little traffic. They both inhale fumes from all of the traffic on Main Street but about 20% of what Patty is taking in. By 6:45 am, they both are back home ready for a quick shower. So far they have only had one exposure of any appreciable amount.

Both of them understand that the water supply is somewhat tainted but neither is willing to shell out the big bucks to have an expensive filtration system that would also remove most of the chemicals from their bath and shower water. They hop in the shower and get exposed to the same chemicals Patty and Donny did. Two more exposures for our healthy couple.

What is different though is the shampoos and conditioners they use. They went to the Environmental Working Groups website, www.ewg.org and found the article entitled "Skin Deep". They found the least toxic shampoos and conditioners and use them instead of the ones laden with toxins.

From here Bernice and Stan have breakfast, which varies from day to day. Sometimes it is leftover fish from the night before (wild, not farmed), or it could be a couple of organically grown eggs and some whole wheat toast. They have learned from experience that the wider the variety of foods one eats, the healthier you become.

Both Bernice and Stan are high-powered executives but they try to work within some limits to avoid over-stressing themselves. They like to get to work early, but they do it when necessary and not all the time. They take vacations each year (no building it up like Patty and Donny) to make sure they take care of their bodies.

Also, they have incorporated a simple nutritional supplement regime which looks like this:

- A multi-vitamin/multi-mineral pack
- One gram of high quality omega 3 fish oils tested for toxins.
- A high potency probiotic.
- One gram of taurine and a 50mg CoEnzyme Q10 supplement.
- A carnitine supplement (500 mg) with biotin.
- Stan has an extra capsule of magnesium (250 mg) as men have a greater need for this mineral.
- They also take a capsule of the herb Milk Thistle to support their liver (the bodies main detox unit).
- And they wash it all down with some filtered water mixed with high quality electrolytes.

Both couples try their best to do what is right, Bernice and Stan just do it smarter. When we look at both couples we see that small differences in their actions can make a difference. It becomes bigger when we realize that these habits occur everyday and when you multiply the exposures over a ten year period you can see how the probabilities of getting a serious disease is far greater for Pat and Don over Bernice and Stan. If Pat is exposed to sixteen toxins each morning and you multiply that by 365 days over ten years you get a staggering, 58,400 exposures in the morning alone! Bernice, if she gets exposed six times each morning, she gets 21,900 times (which is still an amazing amount). If you remember my loaded revolver theory chapter you can see how the additional 36,500 exposures can load the chambers of the toxic gun up real fast.

Bottom line is if you, as a concerned individual, can lower the number of toxic exposures you and your family face by say six each day, over a five year period you will lower the number times you absorb a toxin 10,950 times. Think long and hard about that and realize how easy that is.

15. A Little Ditty, a Little Humor

"To appreciate nonsense requires a serious interest in life."

Gelett Burgess

"Anyone who takes himself too seriously always runs the risk of looking ridiculous; anyone who can consistently laugh at himself does not."

Vaclav Havel

"Music is a beautiful opiate, if you don't take it too seriously."

Henry Miller

We all need a little fun in our lives. This is especially true when talking about as heavy a subject as environmental toxicity. Here is my attempt to bring a little humor into everyone's life.

Music and song has been shown to hit at people's emotions better than almost anything else. So for our brief interlude I bring you a little ditty I wrote late one night when nothing else would come to mind. It is to be sung to the tune of Strangers in the Night made famous by the late, great singer Frank Sinatra (my apologies to him).

TOXINS IN THE NIGHT

Toxins in the night, inhaling gases
Phthalates in my Sprite
We're taking chances
We'd be sharing coughs
Before the night was through.

Toxins in your eyes so irritating,
Toxins in your smile so darned inflaming,
Toxins in my heart,
Gave me angina toooooooo.

Toxins in the night, two wheezing people
We were eating toxins in the night
Up to the moment
When we said our first achooo.
Little did we know
Asthma was just a glance away,
A warm and mucous hack away and -

Ever since that night we've been together.
Wheezers at first sight, in detox forever.
It turned out so right,
For toxins in the night.

16. Obesity and Toxicity–It's not just McDonald's fault

"Thou seest I have more flesh than another man, and therefore more frailty."

William Shakespeare

"Now there are more overweight people in America than average-weight people. So overweight people are now average. Which means you've met your New Year's resolution."

Jay Leno

"Imprisoned in every fat man is a thin one wildly signaling to be let out."

Cyril Connolly

It seems that every day you read another story about the obesity epidemic in America. You go to the local book store and the most popular part is the diet section. Atkins, South Beach, Blood Type, Pritikin, Glycemic Index, and on and on. The truth be known, most only work for about 10-20% of the people who actually use them and most often, only for the short term. So why is it so hard to lose weight and more importantly, keep it off?

In 2002, while working with a dear friend who was also the head of nutrition for a prestigious cancer clinic, I came up with an answer (not *the* answer, no one has that) and it was toxicity. Of this issue, I could (and probably will) right an entire book, but in this setting I will go over my assumptions briefly.

In animal studies there is an observation usually made that as a laboratory rat is exposed to toxins, their metabolic rate drops and their internal temperature goes down as well. As you can imagine, this phenomena occurs in humans as well. As you have seen in previous chapters, we have been increasing the body load of toxicity in people every year and with so many of us having impaired detoxification pathways, it would seem that body temperatures would follow the pattern exhibited by animal studies.

Guess what? The pattern fits. A few years ago, the American Medical Association debated whether to drop the average healthy body temperature of patients from 98.6 degrees Fahrenheit to 98.0 degrees not because it was healthier to be lower but because fewer and fewer people were coming into doctor's offices with the higher temperature. So instead of trying to figure out why this was happening, they just moved the norm down. Kind of like the Jay Leno quote at the top of the page.

What is the mechanism behind this temperature drop and what is its implication in the obesity explosion? First off, I believe that toxins affect the main cellular energy producing pathway known as the Citric Acid Cycle (aka TCA Cycle or Kreb's Cycle). From observations I have seen in the results from urinary organic acid tests, I believe that toxins, ranging from heavy metals to petrochemical solvents actually block the entry point into the cycle, primarily stunting the ability of the body to produce energy from carbohydrates. This inhibition I believe causes a slowdown in our bodies' resting metabolism.

Here is how it slowly makes us gain weight. First off, not all of the energy we expend is when we are active; our bodies still need energy to keep our systems going. Suppose we ingest 2,500 calories and our daily activities use up 25% of our intake or 625 of those calories, the remainder of the calories that need to be burned equals 1875. In a normal (if that even exists today) person, they would burn those last 1875 calories while at rest. In a toxic person, my estimate is that their chemical load impairs their caloric burn by about 7%. One-hundred and thirty one calories remain unburned which in turn gets stored. Do this for one year and you get 47,815 calories left behind (365 days X 131 calories). Typically if you burn 3,500 calories you lose one pound. Take those 47,815 calories and divide this by 3,500 and you get 13.66 pounds worth of weight gain a year. Do that for 10 years and you have increased your weight by 136.6 pounds and you are now officially obese.

What if my theory only causes the system to lose only 2% efficiency or 37.5 calories a day? Using the same math you would be storing 13,688 calories a year or the equivalent of 3.9 pounds a year. In 10 years you will have gained 39 pounds, and that would increase your risk for a number of diseases and lower your life expectancy. Add to this the fact that many Americans do not exercise and you can see why so many people are walking around with 50 to 100 pounds of excess weight.

In a presentation given at BoulderFest 2006 by Dr. Stefan Siebrecht, citing research done by Berg, et al (2005) he showed that exercise does not help lose weight in most people but only helps to not gain any pounds. This is somewhat profound and makes you realize that if someone truly wants to lose weight it is by improving the resting metabolic rate that you can hope to succeed. Since Dr. Siebrecht calculates that from 60-75% of the day's energy production is at rest (and by rest we mean not exercising or physically exerting oneself), if toxins can (and they do) impair this process, we need to discover ways to improve that mechanism through detoxification and toxin avoidance.

Another mechanism involved in obesity and the inability to lose weight was theorized by a team of researchers led by Dr. Angelo Tremblay of the University of Laval and published in the International Journal of Obesity and Related Metabolic Disorders.[43] In the article, the researchers believe that as people lose weight, the concentration of the toxins go up (the total amount of toxins stays the same) which reduces thermogensis, thereby slowing down or stopping the continuation of weight loss. What this means is that in order to have a long term successful weight loss program, we need to help the individual detoxify simultaneously.

At one of my lectures, a physician asked me whether it would not be simpler to just increase an obese person's metabolism instead of worrying about the theoretical effects of toxicity. My answer was to think about why the body lowers its metabolism and temperature. The reason for it is to reduce the effects of the incoming or existing toxins, and so by increasing metabolism you would be doing harm to the individual. His response surprised me. The doctor said that if I was right, by adding thyroid hormones to an individual without assessing their toxicity level he and his colleagues would be doing something potentially dangerous. I nodded my head in affirmation.

Millions of people on thyroid medications would be wise to assess their toxic load through appropriate laboratory testing as they may be doing themselves a great deal of harm. If toxins are evident, then a detoxification protocol through an educated practitioner may help reduce the need for thyroid medications (whether synthetic or natural). If your physician is thinking of putting you on thyroid meds without testing for environmental toxicity then you may need to do some exploring on your own and find a practitioner willing to look at this potential avenue of treatment.

Another mechanism by which certain toxins affect weight is how many of them cause impairment of the human endocrine system. This includes the pancreas and the way you deal with insulin and blood sugar, the thyroid which helps regulate metabolism, the adrenals, the pituitary and the master control organ, the hypothalamus. Toluene, a common petrochemical solvent, has been shown to cause dysfunction in the hypothalamus which can cause the rest of the endocrine system to malfunction.[44]

In a study published in October 2004, researchers led by Tian Xia from UCLA showed that quinones and other aromatic chemicals as well as ultrafine particles can severely interfere with the ability of mitochondria to produce energy. Not only that, they reported that some chemicals cause mitochondrial bloating, structural decomposition, increased production of free radicals, and cellular apoptosis (cell death/suicide).[45] If the chemicals in question came in on small particles they were better able to penetrate cell walls, thereby wrecking more havoc within the cell.

There is one more issue relating to obesity and that is the correlation between it and diabetes. Most people who read the news have seen numerous medical reports linking the two conditions to the point that it is accepted as gospel. Guess what? It may not be as definitive as you think.

Turns out that the relationship between obesity and diabetes has a third player involved, toxicity, in the form of persistent organic pollutants known as POPs.[46] This family of toxins includes DDT, dioxin, PCBs and chlordane. A few studies have shown that obese people who had detectable levels of POPs were far more likely to develop diabetes than those who had undetectable levels. The Korean study led by Dr. DH Lee showed that the increased risk of developing diabetes when all six of the studied toxins were found in a person was thirty-eight fold. This number is absolutely staggering. This is yet another reason to make sure that you detoxify yourself and prevent exposure to these chemicals.

As I said before, this subject is a lot more complicated than this brief chapter can cover, but I truly believe that not only are our diets to blame for the growing obesity epidemic but that toxicity does not only add to the problem but it makes the solution ever so much more difficult to achieve. Considering that in 1995, the estimated cost of obesity in the United States was $99.5 billion dollars a year and that the rate of obesity has climbed rapidly since then, it would not be out of the question to figure that the economic expense of obesity was probably over $150 billion dollars in 2006.[47] Given this drain on the economy and the enormous human cost, we should begin to realize that the abuse we have heaped on our environment is effecting our own survival and needs to be dealt with before it is too late.

Our children, and subsequently their children, will look at us with disgust when they realize why they are as obese as they are with no way out. The time is now to make the changes necessary to save ourselves and our world.

In most books, this is where the author would dazzle you with a series of recommendations that would help you increase your metabolic rate and detoxify you. They would list a series of nutrients, diets, protocols or whatever suited their fancy. Sorry, but this writer would not be doing that today.

Why not you might ask? The reason is simple. You are all biochemically different and there are no universal answers to the issue of toxicity. It is not like giving you a food recipe to follow. No one knows what your true lifetime exposure to toxins has been. We cannot guess at the capacity of your body to excrete the multitude of chemicals. Is your gut full of pathogenic bacteria that can transform beneficial amino acids into a potentially toxic phenol compound? The only way to get around this dilemma is to test each person and then treat them in a biochemically individualized manner and slowly and carefully help them detoxify and increase their metabolic rate safely.

17. TOXINS IN OUR ENVIRONMENT

"The poor trend lightest on the earth. The higher our income, the more resources we control and the more havoc we wreak."

Paul Harrison

"I am I plus my surroundings and if I do not preserve the latter, I do not preserve myself."

Jose Ortega Y Gassett

"The new American finds his challenge and his love in the traffic-chocked streets, skies nested in smog, choking with the acids of industry, the screech of rubber and houses leashed in against one another while the townlets wither a town and die."

John Stienbeck

While not a complete discussion of the numerous toxins in this chapter and certainly not a complete listing of all of the toxins in our environment, these are, in my opinion the most important to understand. As the old saying goes, know your enemies to best learn how to defeat them.

ARSENIC

A legendary poison, this heavy metal is naturally occurring but it is still considered a very toxic element with the inorganic form being more toxic than the organic form. Arsenic is typically found combined with one or more other elements such as oxygen, chlorine and sulfur. For centuries, it was used as a medicine in the treatment of diseases such as syphilis and amoebic dysentery as well as other infections.[48]

Most of the arsenic found in our environment (74%) comes from the use of a wood preservative, chromated copper arsenate, which was phased out of use in the United States in 2002 and eliminated worldwide on December 31, 2003. While its continued application has been stopped, the sheer volume of its use in the past it will cause it to remain a problem for many decades as it leeches from the pressure treated wood and finds its way to our top soil and eventually to underground aquifers and our water supply.

Arsenic is also used in insecticides, weed killers, fungicides (19%), glass production (3%), semiconductors, and some medications typically used in chicken feed to control parasites. The process of making metal alloys such as lead buckshot also involves the use of arsenic. A full 70% of the exposure of arsenic by weight is through our food supply, mostly as the organic form. The inorganic, and more toxic, form is found predominantly in water (29%).

COMMON FORMS:

- chromated copper arsenate (CCA)
- arsenic pentoxide
- calcium arsenate
- lead arsenate
- sodium arsenate
- arsenic trioxide
- potassium arsenate

HEALTH EFFECTS:

- Extremely toxic if inhaled or ingested, very toxic if absorbed through skin.
- Known carcinogen, especially lung cancer.
- Endocrine disruptor. Inhaled arsenic may cause irritation to the lungs and throat, may damage blood vessels, cause depression of red blood cell production, and cause an abnormal heart rhythm. Skin redness and dryness is another possible sign of arsenic poisoning.

Longer term exposure is often followed by symptoms of fatigue and malaise along with gastrointestinal distress, anemia, skin disruptions including spots on the skin, pale bands on the fingernails and toes, hyperkeratosis, and "pins and needles" sensation in hands and feet. Laboratory tests for arsenic in hair, nails, and urine may be present long after exposure has stopped while fecal metal tests are more likely to show high while being exposed.

As with many toxins a link has been shown between arsenic exposure and immunological and cardiovascular disease, including hypertension, coronary artery disease, peripheral vascular disease, and atherosclerosis. Type II diabetes has also been seen in studies of arsenic poisoning.

Individuals with low protein diets or choline deficiency may be more sensitive to arsenic than the general population. In addition, people with low dietary folate (folic acid) are more susceptible to arsenic's toxic effects.[49]

EXPOSURE PATHWAYS/SOURCES:

Children chewing on arsenic treated wood as well as when they touch the wood and put their hands in their mouths are two major sources of exposure. Playing in soil contaminated where the treated wood has leeched its arsenic is another way to be exposed.[50]

Inhalation of arsenic is normally found in areas where arsenic was used industrially or when arsenic treated wood was being cut (sawdust).

The highest levels of arsenic in our diets are found in seafood, poultry, mushrooms, salt, and grains. Non-organically grown chicken typically has the highest levels of arsenic because of the drugs used to control parasites contains this heavy metal.[51] Seafood contains the organic form of arsenic, which is typically less toxic.

Drinking water from the tap in areas (especially the southeast U.S.) with high concentrations of arsenic is another source of ingestion.[52]

MISCELLANEOUS COMMENTS:

- Industrial release of arsenic was estimated to be 12 billion pounds in 1999 according to the Environmental Protection Agency.[53]
- Drinking water exposes an estimated 11 million Americans.[54]
- Low levels of arsenic may disrupt the endocrine system.[55]
- All production of arsenic is from outside the United States.

TOP 5 STATES WITH THE HIGHEST OUTPUT OF ARSENIC IN THE U.S.

Nevada - 63,103,035 pounds
South Dakota - 9,900,619
California - 2,352,017
Idaho - 647,526
Texas - 402,817

LABORATORY TESTING:

- Hair Elements – Long-term exposure - Doctor's Data – Most Recommended. Inexpensive and when interpreted properly, filled with valuable information.
- Fecal Metals – Ongoing exposure – Doctor's Data – Best to assess current exposure.
- RBC Mineral Toxin – Ongoing and Long-term exposure – Doctor's Data, MetaMetrix – May be helpful.
- Urine Heavy Metals – Ongoing and Long-term exposure – Doctor's Data – Used with DMSA or DMPS challenges (not recommended by this author).

Benzene

Known as an aromatic hydrocarbon and a volatile organic compound (VOC), which easily releases fumes, benzene is a very common toxin found predominantly in industrial applications and not in common household products.

Benzene is used as a major building block in the manufacturing of industrial chemicals, plastics, rubber, resins, synthetic fabrics, dyes, detergents and explosives.

The majority of exposure to humans comes in the form of tobacco smoke (predominant), gasoline and automobile exhaust. Other exposure possibilities include: asphalt, pesticides, synthetic rubber and adhesives. Benzene is also used as a solvent in waxes, resins, paints, inks and some craft supplies.

Natural sources of benzene are volcanoes and forest fires (especially pine forests). The benzene ring is also a common component of vitamins, sugars and a number of enzymes. This "ring" is non-toxic though and has no effect on health.

Health Effects:

- Extremely toxic if ingested or inhaled, toxic if absorbed through the skin.
- Carcinogenic, linked to leukemia and blood diseases like multiple myeloma.
- Neurotoxic, especially in cases where the individual has inadequate Phase II detoxification capabilities (low glycine, poor glutathione production).
- Anemia from the loss of red blood cell production, bone marrow damage, excessive bleeding, weakened immune system, drying and scaling of skin.
- Drowsiness, headaches, loss of consciousness are a few of the effects on the central nervous system.
- Respiratory failure can lead to death in extreme cases.
- Chromosomal damage.
- It is believed to cause tumors in animals and possibly in humans.

Exposure Pathways/Sources:

Of all of the exposures benzene fumes can be inhaled from both smoking and in secondhand tobacco smoke, which accounts for an estimated 50% of the public's exposure.[56] One estimate claimed that smokers dump thirty metric tons of benzene into their collective lungs annually. Drinking contaminated water as well as absorbing it through skin while showering are ways to expose oneself to this solvent.

Inhalation of benzene occurs due to living near high traffic areas and while pumping gas, as well as from household automotive and industrial cleaning products, carpet glues, textured carpets and rugs, and furniture waxes (all of which contain small amounts of benzene).

Miscellaneous Comments:

- The annual benzene production in the U.S. was estimated at 2.3 billion gallons in 1997.[57]
- According to the U.S. EPA, approximately 495 million tons of benzene are released into the U.S. environment every year from industrial and pharmaceutical manufacturing plants.[58]
- When using paint thinners, adhesives and harsh chemical containing benzene, make sure the area is well ventilated and that children are not in the area as they are most susceptible to the effects of this toxin due to poor excretion capabilities.[59]
- Benzene is considered one of the 100 most significant hazardous substances as determined by EPA and the Agency for Toxic Substances and Disease Registry.

Laboratory Testing:

- Blood or adipose tissue testing for levels of benzene may be obtained through Accu-Chem Laboratories.
- Urinary metabolites of benzene can be obtained through U.S. Biotek in the Environmental Pollutant Biomarker Tests.

How to Lower Exposure:

- Do not run, jog, or walk near high traffic areas.
- Do not smoke cigarettes and cigars and avoid people who do.
- Reduce the use of benzene containing solvents (it is on the label) and if you do have to use them, ventilate your area well and keep children away.
- Do not run combustion engines indoors.

Bisphenol A

A major building block of polycarbonate plastic, bisphenol A is used to make baby bottles, Nalgene® bottles, and 5-gallon water bottles. The stiffer, larger bottles are made to be sturdier and are more likely to contain bisphenol A versus smaller and more flexible bottles. It is also used in epoxy resins, in the plastic lining of many food cans, dental sealants, and as an additive in other consumer products.

Bisphenol A was originally synthesized in the lab back in 1891 but its estrogenicity (being estrogen like and/or stimulating the production of estrogen) was first discovered in 1936 in studies done by Dodds and Lawson.[60] Soon thereafter it was discovered that this hormone could be polymerized to form polycarbonate plastic. BPA is not stable and will decay over time, releasing it into both food and water despite industry claims to the contrary.

Health Effects:

- Highly toxic if inhaled, ingested or absorbed through skin.
- Can damage male reproductive organs
- Implicated in obesity
- Sperm damage
- Premature puberty
- Down's syndrome
- Multiple birth defects

EXPOSURE PATHWAYS/SOURCES:
- Leeching from polycarbonate baby bottles.
- Leeching from the inner plastic coating used in canned foods.
- Large five gallon water bottles used commonly in office water dispensers have been found to have traces of the toxin.
- Dental sealants.

MISCELLANEOUS COMMENTS:

On average, humans ingest approximately 6.3 micrograms per day of bisphenol-A from the linings of food cans. Bisphenol-A is one of the top 50 chemicals produced in the U.S. Over 1.6 billion pounds of this hormone disruptor were produced in 1995.[61]

LABORATORY TESTING:
- Blood and adipose tissue testing from Accu-Chem Laboratories

HOW TO LOWER EXPOSURE:
- Do not use polycarbonate bottles, especially baby bottles.
- If you use plastic bottles, never heat them, ever, regardless of the type of bottle.
- If your bottles are scratched, throw them away. Again, any type of plastic bottle.
- Choose frozen or fresh foods over canned.

CADMIUM

Cadmium is a naturally occurring heavy metal found in many rocks and soil. It is also used in the manufacture of Teflon® and in fertilizers, and is released from the burning of coal. Batteries contain cadmium as do paints, plastics (primarily polyvinyl chloride - PVC, or vinyl), ceramic glazes, textile dyes and cigarette smoking.

One of the biggest problems with cadmium is how it is gradually building up in our agricultural soils. This contamination is why food contributes 80-90% of the cadmium we receive (non-smokers).

COMMON FORMS:

- cadmium oxide
- cadmium carbonate
- cadmium chloride
- cadmium nitrate
- cadmium sulfide
- cadmium sulfate
- cadmium selenium sulfide
- cadmium telluride

HEALTH EFFECTS:

- Known carcinogen.
- Reproductive and development toxicant.
- May be an endocrine disruptor.
- It has been known to cause lung damage due to inhalation,
- Kidney damage from ingestion
- Can suppress the immune system.
- Linked to multiple cancers such as prostate, kidney and bladder carcinomas in humans.

EXPOSURE PATHWAYS/SOURCES:

- Contaminated water is one way of exposure as it may leach from galvanized zinc pipes.
- It is commonly absorbed through ingestion and inhalation.
- Absorption through the skin is possible but not considered a major exposure risk.
- Solders used in copper piping and the leaching from batteries in landfills into aquifers.
- Young children can also get exposed by chewing on vinyl toys, rain coats, umbrellas, clothing, backpacks, ponchos, school supplies, purses and sports equipment.
- Other sources include glazes for ceramics and glass as well as fabric dyes.
- Shellfish such as shrimp, lobster, clams, oysters, mussels.
- Organ meats like kidney and liver.

- Sunflower seeds.
- Green leafy vegetables, cereal grains, potatoes, and milk.
- Phosphate rich fertilizers used in food production.
- Cigarette smoke, both active and secondhand.

MISCELLANEOUS COMMENTS:

About 25,000 to 30,000 tons of cadmium are released to the environment each year through the normal course of nature, about half occurring from the weathering of rocks into river water and then to the oceans. Forest fires and volcanoes also release some cadmium to the air. Release of cadmium from human activities is estimated to be from 4,000 to 13,000 tons per year, with major contributions from mining and from burning fossil fuels.[62] Food and cigarette smoke are the biggest sources of cadmium exposure for people in the general population.

LABORATORY TESTING:

- Hair Elements – Long-term exposure - Doctor's Data – Most Recommended. Inexpensive and when interpreted properly, filled with valuable information.
- Fecal Metals – Ongoing exposure – Doctor's Data – Best to assess current exposure.
- RBC Mineral Toxin – Ongoing and Long-term exposure – Doctor's Data, MetaMetrix – May be helpful.
- Urine Heavy Metals – Ongoing and Long-term exposure – Doctor's Data – Used with DMSA or DMPS challenges (not recommended by this author).

HOW TO LOWER EXPOSURE:

- Recycle batteries
- If you are using a product with cadmium, make sure you have a mask on and the area is well ventilated.
- Do not smoke and avoid people who do.
- Recycle old computer equipment and other electronic products.
- Install a water filtration/reverse osmosis system in your house if on well water.

DIOXIN

An organochlorine compound, there are currently 75 known forms of dioxin which are byproducts of the manufacturing and use of chlorine. The bleaching of paper and the burning of residential waste add to the atmospheric load of this chemical toxin.

Human exposure comes from the burning of chemicals made of chlorine, including pesticides and PCBs.

Dioxin is a long-lasting chemical which can travel great distances and has been found in the vast majority of mammals, amphibians, reptiles and fish world-wide. Fetal exposure is rampant as are detectable and dangerous levels in human breast milk.

COMMON FORMS:

While there are 75 forms of dioxin, 2,3,7,8-tetrachlorodibenzo-para-dioxin (aka TCDD) is the most toxic and commonly comes from the burning of plastics.

HEALTH EFFECTS:

- Highly carcinogenic.
- A developmental and reproductive toxicant.
- Known endocrine disruptor.
- Implicated as a cause of Type-2 diabetes.[63]
- Causes numerous fetal developmental problems including: reduced viability, low birth weight, structural alterations, growth retardation, and functional alterations, such as effects on thyroid function, neurodevelopmental delays and impaired cognitive ability.

EXPOSURE PATHWAYS/SOURCES:

- The majority of exposure to humans is through their food. Since dioxin tends to accumulate in fat tissue, meat, poultry, egg, dairy, cheese and shellfish have been known to have significant quantities of this toxin.
- Babies receive much of their dioxin exposure from breast milk.

- Dioxin can cross the placental wall so fetuses will be exposed to the mother's accumulated lifetime exposure.
- Inhalation does not seem to be a common exposure pathway.

Miscellaneous Comments:

A young child's intake of dioxins, furans (related compounds) and dioxin-like PCBs are over three times higher as compared to that of an adult, on a body weight basis. Food accounts for 95 percent of human exposure to dioxin. [64] While the production of dioxin has been banned throughout the world, it is considered a POP or persistent organic pollutant as it does not dissipate from the environment once released.

Laboratory Testing:

- Blood and adipose tissue testing from Accu-Chem Laboratories

How to Lower Exposure:

- Find out what the levels are in your home water supply by calling the local water authority, or by having your well water tested.
- Reduce fat rich foods such as beef, butter, cheeses and fatty fish.
- Eat organic foods. While these may not be entirely devoid of dioxin, they generally contain less than non-organic foods.
- Stay away from farm-bred fish. Choose wild caught fish instead, especially salmon.

Lead

Highly toxic, this naturally occurring heavy metal was commonly used in many household products such as paint, gasoline, PVC pipes, ceramic glazes and caulking. These uses were banned in the 1970s but it is still being used in the production of batteries, ammunition, computer monitors and x-ray shields.

Much of the documented neurological damage done by lead is to developing children, especially those who live in poorer neighborhoods. Recently, a paper also suggested that the neurotoxic effects are greater with increased levels of stress.[65]

Greater than 60% of adult human exposure of lead comes from our food with 30% coming from inhalation of contaminated air and 10% from water. For children, a great deal of the exposure is from soil, dust, and lead-based paints still on the wall of many inner-city apartments.

HEALTH EFFECTS:

- It is a known carcinogen
- A known neurotoxin.
- Can harm the reproductive system
- Can cause serious developmental damage.
- Can cause learning disabilities
- Memory loss
- Decreased IQ
- Attention Deficit Disorder (ADD)
- Aggression
- Stunted growth
- Coronary heart disease
- Hypertension
- Seizures
- Decreased appetite
- Cataracts

EXPOSURE PATHWAYS/SOURCES:

- While it is a naturally occurring metal, it is found in a number of products including:
  - ➢ Paints
  - ➢ Gasoline
  - ➢ PVC (vinyl) plastic
  - ➢ Pipes
  - ➢ Ceramic glazes
  - ➢ Caulk

- It is found in the manufacture of
  - ➢ Batteries
  - ➢ Ammunition
  - ➢ Metal products (solder and pipes)
  - ➢ Devices to shield X-rays
  - ➢ Computer monitors to block radiation

MISCELLANEOUS COMMENTS:

Nearly one million children under the age of six have blood lead levels higher than the lead safety threshold of 10 mcg/dL that has been established by the U.S. Centers for Disease Control and Prevention.[66] To this day millions of homes in the United States contain lead paint.[67]

Over 80 percent of all homes built before 1978 in the U.S. have lead-based paint in them. The older the house, the more likely it is to contain lead-based paint and a higher concentration of lead in the paint.[68]

Numerous studies show that every 10 mcg/dL increase of blood lead level results in a 2-7 point decrease in IQ.[69]

LABORATORY TESTING:

- Hair Elements – Long-term exposure - Doctor's Data – Most Recommended. Inexpensive and when interpreted properly, filled with valuable information.
- Fecal Metals – Ongoing exposure – Doctor's Data – Best to assess current exposure.
- RBC Mineral Toxin – Ongoing and Long-term exposure – Doctor's Data, MetaMetrix – May be helpful.
- Urine Heavy Metals – Ongoing and Long-term exposure – Doctor's Data – Used with an EDTA challenge (not recommended by this author).

MERCURY

Mercury may be the most toxic of all of the heavy metals. It is a definitive neurotoxin, especially for children. The damage, if not treated early on, may cause irreparable neurological damage. The amount of mercury being found in today's environment is staggering. Elemental mercury is found in so many products being dumped into our landfills where it is converted into the more dangerous methylmercury which the entire earth is being polluted with it.

Polar bears are the land mammals with the highest detectable levels of mercury. This is both from dietary sources (fish) and atmospheric (mercury tends to drop out of the atmosphere at the coldest temperatures).

Because liquid mercury vaporizes very quickly it is critical that you proceed with extra caution if you break a mercury containing thermometer (better yet, if you have one, bring it to a hazardous waste dump site in your community) as airborne mercury is more hazardous than liquid.

COMMON FORMS:

- Methylmercury
- Elemental mercury
- Ethylmercury
- Mercuric chloride
- Mercurous chloride
- Metal amalgams (dental fillings)

HEALTH EFFECTS:

This section can quickly turn into a book. The health effects of even the smallest amounts of mercury are truly frightening. Everything from cancer to cardiovascular disease, autism to epilepsy, birth defects to developmental damage, this heavy metal's exposure needs to be avoided at all costs.

While industry spokespeople claim that small amounts are harmless, when exposed to as many sources as modern humans are, this is a smokescreen and down right deceitful. On top of that, there are a number of people who have a genetic inability to excrete even small amounts of mercury (Apolipoprotein E3/E4 or E4/E4).

High doses can cause permanent damage and in some cases death. Of course, the definition of high dose with mercury can vary from tens to hundreds of micrograms depending on the individual.

Exposure Pathways/Sources:

- Vaccines (thimerasol)
- Fish and Seafood
- Dental Amalgams
- Fluorescent light bulbs
- Energy Efficient light bulbs (although much less than earlier models)
- Electrical switches
- Multimineral supplements that claim high numbers of minerals and come from so-called "natural" sources may have traces of mercury
- Coal burning plants
- Waste dumps, especially capped ones
- The Great Salt Lake and other waterways near mining operations
- Old gas meters

Miscellaneous Comments:

The issue of mercury and human health is a volatile one. On one side are the industrial users who are reluctant to reduce, and then eliminate mercury from their products because of cost. On the other side are the countless millions of people who are suffering from the adverse health effects of mercury, many without ever knowing. It is my strong opinion that every effort must be made to reduce all man-made sources of mercury as fast as possible.

Laboratory Testing:

- Hair Elements – Long-term exposure - Doctor's Data – Most Recommended. Inexpensive and when interpreted properly, filled with valuable information.
- Fecal Metals – Ongoing exposure – Doctor's Data – Best to assess current exposure.
- RBC Mineral Toxin – Ongoing and Long-term exposure – Doctor's Data, MetaMetrix – May be helpful.
- Urine Heavy Metals – Ongoing and Long-term exposure – Doctor's Data – Used with DMSA or DMPS challenges (not recommended by this author).

PARABENS

Long considered safe, parabens are being increasingly investigated as a potential carcinogen, endocrine disruptor and hormone mimicker. While extremely small scale, the study linking this toxin found mostly in cosmetics, anti-perspirants and deodorants to an increased risk of breast cancer is quite disturbing.

COMMON FORMS:

- Ethylparaben
- Methylparaben
- Butylparaben
- Propylparaben

HEALTH EFFECTS:

The field of paraben toxicity is only now being seriously studied as they have always been considered GRAS (generally regarded as safe) but recent studies have suggested that this may not be the case. A recent 2004 paper suggests that parabens may be implicated in breast cancer.[70,71] Other possible issues that have been suggested include endocrine disruption and hormone mimickery.[72]

EXPOSURE PATHWAYS:

There are two primary exposure pathways for parabens
- Eating processed food[73] sometimes contain parabens without having it on the label.
- Absorbing it through the skin via skin care products.[74] Go to www.ewg.org for the report "Skin Deep" for further information.

MISCELLANEOUS COMMENTS:

While not the most toxic of substances in this list, it is one of the most common. My concerns with parabens are not with them alone, but as another additive that stacks the deck against our abilities to achieve optimal health.

LABORATORY TESTING:

- Blood and adipose tissue testing from Accu-Chem Laboratories
- Urinary metabolite testing from U.S. Biotek

PERCHLORATES

This almost ubiquitous chemical is the most oxidized salt of the chlorooxyacids. It is predominantly used as a fuel oxidizer for rockets and missiles. While there are few launches of rockets using perchlorates, the amount used for one space shuttle launch is a staggering 350,000 kilograms.[75] Considering that the EPA set a standard (which many of us think is somewhat high) of 24.5 parts per *billion*, Theo Colborn, author of "*Our Stolen Future*" has spent the past decade warning people of the potential dangers of pervasiveness of perchlorates in our environment.[76] Recent research has suggested that this chemical can negatively affect thyroid function in both men and women.[77]

COMMON FORMS:

- potassium perchlorate
- ammonium perchlorate
- sodium perchlorate
- magnesium perchlorate

HEALTH EFFECTS:

Aside from its ability to inhibit iodine uptake to the thyroid gland, the most disturbing problem with this toxin is its alleged disruption in fetal development and neurological damage done to children.[78] Even at levels as low as parts per billion or trillion, the effects on a developing child are devastating. Aside from neurological damage, sexual development may also be impaired. Of course industry scientists may rail against some of this data but my belief is that they do so because they view their responsibility for the totality of the issue as ending with their chemical alone and not the cumulative effect of all of the other hormone disruptors and the like. When you add to the mix all of the other ubiquotos chemicals into a developing fetus, we get a chemical soup that can severely disrupt their development and therefore their future.

EXPOSURE PATHWAYS:

Most of the exposure, short of living near a rocket launching facility is through the drinking of perchlorate polluted water. You can find out if you live in an area that may have perchlorates (along with many other pollutants) in the water by going to www.scorecard.org.

MISCELLANEOUS COMMENTS:

Most research into perchlorates has been done to determine their LD50 level, the level at which 50% of the tested animals die.

According to the paper "Body Burden" by the Environmental Working Group (www.ewg.org) "A growing body of literature links low dose chemical exposures in animal studies to a broad range of health effects previously unexplored in high dose studies."[79]

With some chemicals, an effect seen at a high dose is not seen at a low dose and visa versus. Perchlorate, a rocket fuel component, causes changes in the brain at .01 – 1 mg/kg per day but not at 30 mg/kg per day according to Argus 1998 and others. We see with perchlorates that an effect seen at a low dose does not appear at a higher dose. This effect is known as a biphasic dose response.[80] This phenomena is not well understood but is seen often in biochemistry.

Most importantly, in an issue of Environmental Health Perspectives, 2004, the following statements were made: "...there is broad agreement that perchlorate interferes with the uptake of iodine into the thyroid gland as well as other tissues, including the placenta and mammary gland.... Whereas adults have the reserve capacity to withstand a month or more with limited iodine intake, a fetus or infant can be harmed much more rapidly due to the reliance of the developing brain on adequate thyroid hormone levels."[81]

LABORATORY TESTING:

- Blood and adipose tissue testing from Accu-Chem Laboratories

Phthalates

Phthalates are plasticizers used in the manufacturing of polyvinyl chloride (PVC, vinyl) products which include children's toys, building products such as plastic water pipes, and medical tubing. It is also found in a number of personal care products such as shampoos, conditioners, cosmetics, air fresheners, scented candles, time-released medications and supplements. Phthalates are used in many products to hold scents and aromas.

Common Forms:

- DEHP - Di(2-ethylhexyl)phthalate
- DINP - diisononyl phthalate
- DBP - di-n-butyl phthalate
- DEP - Diethyl Phthalate
- DIP - diisodecyl phthalate

Health Effects:

- Some forms of phthalates have been shown to be carcinogenic.
- Birth defects such as cleft palate and underdeveloped male reproductive organs have been seen in both humans and animals.
- Premature breast development in young girls have been seen directly proportional to blood concentrations.
- Potentially interferes with testosterone.
- Damages the DNA in male sperm.
- Has been implicated in increased waist circumference in men.
- May cause insulin resistance and weight gain in males.

Exposure Pathways:

- Inhalation from air fresheners, scented candles and from new cars outgassing (when the plastics in the car breakdown).
- Ingestion from time-released medications and nutritional supplements.

- Intravenously from plastic blood bags and IVs using plastic medical tubing.
- Inhalation from perfumes, nail polish and other scented products.
- Skin absorption from skin moisturizers, shampoos and conditioners.

MISCELLANEOUS COMMENTS:

Because of its ability to affect fetal development this is a chemical that needs banning. We are still learning about all of the potential side effects of this ubiquitous toxin but one thing we do know is that it needs to be kept far away from children and pregnant women as much as possible. Recent research has suggested that the effects on males may be significant, especially how phthalates may thyroid function[82] and insulin resistance[83].

The most important message I can give you here is to avoid microwaving food in plastic containers or wrapped in plastic wrap, do not buy plastic shower curtains (try cloth instead), and avoid foam-filled furniture. If you buy these products, manufacturers will continue making them. When you throw phthalate containing plastics away the problem does not go away with it. Phthalates will leach into the groundwater and into the air through outgassing. My advice is to find alternatives whenever possible.

LABORATORY TESTING:

- Blood and adipose tissue testing from Accu-Chem Laboratories
- Urinary metabolite testing from U.S. Biotek

POLYCHLORINATED BIPHENYLS (PCBS)

Polychlorinated biphenyls are a group of chemicals that are known as organochlorine compounds. While these chemicals were banned in the U.S. in 1977, they still persist in our environment due to illegal or improper dumping of products that contained PCBs. In 1970, the estimated production of PCBs topped 85 million pounds so we are talking about a substantial toxic legacy here.

Considered a persistent organic pollutant (POP), PCBs stay in the environment and in humans as well as animals for long periods of time as well as traveling globally from their place of origin. Tests indicate that women's breast milk is often times contaminated with PCBs as well as being found in most people's blood. Areas such as the Hudson River in New York as well as Lake Michigan have had warnings issued to any one thinking of consuming fish from these waterways because of PCB contamination.

Health Effects:

- A known carcinogen
- Strong neurotoxin
- Has been shown to interfere with fetal and child development
- Is commonly thought to be an endocrine disruptor

Exposure Pathways/Sources:

- Food is a major source of PCBs especially those with high levels of fat including oily fish, meat, dairy products and coastal seafood. The higher up in the food chain an animal or fish is, the more likely they are to contain PCBs.
- Breast milk has been found to be contaminated with this toxin.
- Landfills
- Drinking water
- Old houses constructed before 1977 may have remnants of products that once used PCBs

Miscellaneous Comments:

PCBs can accumulate in fish to levels up to more than one million times the concentration in the surrounding water.[84]

Laboratory Testing:

- Blood and adipose tissue testing from Accu-Chem Laboratories

Styrene

Styrene is one of those toxins that seem to be everywhere. It is a byproduct of automobile exhaust, so high-traffic areas create the highest exposure problems. Because it is found in so many products it is found commonly in air, water and soil. While many view styrene as a milder toxin that others, we cannot forget that toxicology is still learning about the cumulative and synergistic effects of chemical toxins and that styrene may be more toxic than is generally thought.

Common Forms:

- Styrofoam
- Polystyrene
- Solvents
- Most paints
- Epoxy resins

Health Effects:

- Styrene is considered a possible carcinogen
- It is a neurotoxin
- It is commonly thought to be an endocrine disruptor

Exposure Pathways/Sources:

- You are not going to believe this one but styrene is used in small quantities as a flavoring agent in some candies and ice cream.
- Some water supplies have trace amounts of styrene.
- Styrofoam cups, food containers (especially meats, fish and poultry)
- Car and truck exhaust
- Paints, varnishes and adhesives
- Cigarette smoke, both active and secondhand.

Miscellaneous Comments:

Styrene was detected in 100% of people studied in a 1982 survey of human fat tissue conducted by the Environmental Protection Agency.[85]

In 1993, over 10 billion pounds of styrene were produced in the U.S. It is the most active generator of smog in the atmosphere. U.S. industrial output in 1998 was 56 million pounds, mostly released into the air.

In reviewing the data from thousands of urinary excretion tests for solvents, I have noticed that most test results come back with some level of styrene excretion. The two markers are mandelic acid (mandelate) and phenylglyoxcilic acid (phenylglyoxylate). When both appear elevated, it is a clear indicator of styrene exposure which should make the person tested review their habits and lower their contact with this toxin.

LABORATORY TESTING:

- Blood and adipose tissue testing from Accu-Chem Laboratories
- Urinary metabolite testing from U.S. Biotek

TOLUENE

A sweet-smelling solvent, toluene is found in hundreds of consumer and industrial products from adhesives to nail polish, cosmetics to paints and paint thinners as well as in gasoline exhaust and cigarette smoke.

It is produced in petroleum refining as a byproduct of styrene manufacturing and is used to produce benzene and urethane. One of the main reasons toluene use has increased is that it replaced lead as a gasoline additive (along with benzene and other aromatic hydrocarbons) to increase octane ratings and reduce engine knocking.[86]

HEALTH EFFECTS:

- It is not considered to be a known carcinogen but it is suspected of being such.
- It is considered to be a neurotoxin.
- It is a documented endocrine disruptor especially to the hypothalamus.
- It is also been shown to interfere with fetal and childhood development.
- May cause kidney and/or liver damage due to long-term exposure.

Exposure Pathways/Sources:

- Most exposures are from inhaling products such as paint, paint thinners, rubber cement, nail polishes, perfumes, stain removers, dyes, inks and adhesives.
- Cigarette smoke, both active and second-hand.
- Car and truck exhaust, especially if you live near a high traffic area.
- Some drinking waters contain toluene but since public water systems are routinely monitored, the only likely source would be unregulated well-water.

Miscellaneous Comments:

Read labels and be aware of the numerous sources of toluene. If you must use it indoors, make sure the area is very well ventilated and no children are around. To find lists of products containing this toxin, go to the National Library of Medicine's Household Products Database at http://householdproducts.nlm.nih.gov/. It is also possible to find toluene free nail polishes, just go to your local health food store and read the labels.

The United States produces about three million tons of toluene annually which represents between one-third and one-quarter of the world's production.[87]

Laboratory Testing:

- Blood and adipose tissue testing from Accu-Chem Laboratories
- Urinary metabolite testing from U.S. Biotek

Xylene

Xylene is an extremely common solvent found in paints, paint thinners, shellacs, lacquers, permanent ink markers, carpet adhesives, rust preventives, nail polish, air fresheners, degreasing cleaners, cigarette smoke and car exhaust. It is also commonly used as the "inert" base for many pesticide solutions.

COMMON FORMS:

- M-xylene
- O-xylene
- P-xylene

HEALTH EFFECTS:

- While no definitive evidence has been published proving the carcinogenicity of xylene, it is likely to cause cancer.
- It is a definitive neurotoxin.
- It also has been shown to interfere with fetal and childhood development.
- Can cause dizziness, headache, fatigue, tremors, memory loss, unconsciousness, and in high enough doses, death.
- Eye, ear and throat irritation is common.
- Can cause birth defects
- Cleft palate, delayed development, and reduced fetus weight may occur in unborn children.
- Also there is an increased risk for miscarriage.

EXPOSURE PATHWAYS/SOURCES:

- Most exposure is through inhalation from car, truck and airplane exhaust as well as gasoline fumes.
- Cigarette smoke, both active and secondhand.
- Inhaling the fumes from paints, paint thinners, varnishes, shellacs, adhesives, permanent ink markers, and rust preventives.
- Water sources that are not regulated have a higher risk of containing xylene.

MISCELLANEOUS COMMENTS:

Xylene is one of the most common chemicals by volume in the United States (top 30). It is estimated that over 600,000 tons are released in the atmosphere annually in the U.S. alone. This solvent is also one of the leading causes of smog.

Alcohol ingestion should be avoided at all costs if you are exposed to xylene as it will inhibit the body's ability to detoxify.[88]

LABORATORY TESTING:

- Blood and adipose tissue testing from Accu-Chem Laboratories
- Urinary metabolite testing from U.S. Biotek

18. TWISTED RESEARCH– TODAY'S WORLD OF MEDICINE

"After all, the ultimate goal of all research is not objectivity, but truth."

Helene Deutsch

"Whenever, therefore, people are deceived and form opinions wide of the truth, it is clear that the error has slid into their minds through the medium of certain resemblances to that truth."

Socrates

"Health is a state of complete physical, mental and social well-being, and not merely the absence of disease or infirmity."

Constitution, The World Health Organization.

With all of my talk about toxicity and the overwhelming evidence that it plays a major role in the etiology of disease and chronic health disorders you would think that modern medicine would focus on it and develop a myriad of treatments to combat the effect of toxins. Obviously, this is not the case. What we have built in our supposedly advanced society is a system of "crutch creation", or symptom treatment protocols without any mind to causation aside from some utterly simplistic recommendations like stop smoking, cut down on your alcohol consumption, exercise and eat according to the food pyramid or whatever the latest, unattainable dietary recommendation from the American Dietetic Association.

Americans as a whole seem to be wholly unwilling to change behavior patterns that lead to ill health and prefer to take a pill to alleviate their ailments. While I am critical of the pharmaceutical industry and their immoral marketing of drugs, they are simply selling into a niche (admittedly a large one) of laziness and lack of responsibility. There isn't as big a market in detoxification and treatment of causation of disease. While the nutritional supplement and health food industry sells somewhere around $23 billion dollars of products a year (includes organic foods, supplements and herbs), the pharmaceutical giant Pfizer did more in 2002 *by itself*!! As you shall see in the next few chapters, the total dollar sales of prescription and non-prescription drugs are absolutely mind boggling.

So the question begs, how did we go so far away from reality? The next two chapters hope to answer that question somewhat by looking at how researchers no longer look at disease using the scientific method but follow the lead of the marketing and financial people running medicine today.

The measurement of uric acid is one of the better single variable test results in assessing the risk of developing coronary health disease, especially hypertension[89] (although there is a lot of debate).[90] Basically, the higher the uric acid, the greater the risk for having a heart attack. A simple and straight forward correlation. So, if we want to lower our chances of having a coronary event (I love euphemisms that soften language), it would make sense to lower uric acid levels, right?

Au contraire mon capitain! If you do that you may increase your risk of developing coronary heart disease. HUH?!?

Let's first understand what uric acid really is. It is a natural defense mechanism, an antioxidant that we produce (many of us do this easily) in times of oxidative stress. Coronary heart disease is likely to be a by-product of an inflammatory process brought on by an increase of oxidative stress over a long period of time. As our abilities to fight off oxidation decrease, or we are accumulating toxins, we need to call on other defense mechanisms such as uric acid to stem the tide (there are other antioxidants we produce but we'll discuss them later).

The theory goes that if we treat someone strictly for gout (a symptomatic sign of elevated uric acid) are we doing the wrong thing and increasing the risk of a heart attack? Unless we have the person change their diet and reduce the known risk factors for CHD along with the treatment (gout is quite painful and sometimes debilitating), we may indeed be doing the exact opposite of what we intended. It's a tough premise to test but the theory remains.

Nutritionally, there are some treatments which work well with dietary changes. First off, people with gout or elevated uric acid need to decrease their intake of refined carbohydrates (everyone should do this), saturated fats and excessive protein. Yes, those of you on Atkins-like diets have an increased incidence of gout (surprise, surprise). Secondly, a broad spectrum of antioxidants would be the next step, with some caution. There is some evidence, although controversial (although not in my opinion – it doesn't happen), that excessive vitamin C in patients with elevated uric acid levels may lead to the formation of kidney stones.[91] The crucial issue is what should be considered excessive in one patient may be low or normal in another. Application of biochemical individuality through the proper use of laboratory testing is called for here.

Another nutritional treatment with some benefit to excessive uric acid is somewhat counterintuitive and that is glycine and amino acids. Hyperuremia is typically found in people with high protein intake and since glycine is a component of proteins you would think this wouldn't work but there is evidence that purine-free amino acid therapy does work at lowering uric acid from the system.[92]

Glycine, as you shall see later in the book, is a wonderful amino acid which is capable of binding to a number of toxins as well as being a component of the tri-peptide antioxidant extraordinaire, glutathione.

There may be another explanation as to why it has been shown to be helpful in treating gout and elevated uric acid levels.

Imagine if you will, adding a gram of glycine (500 mg morning and evening) to your daily regimen. By doing so, you have improved your ability to detoxify a number of solvents which in turn may help to lower your oxidative stress which in turn would lower the need for antioxidants. This would then signal the body that it could lower production of uric acid as the oxidative stress caused by the toxins is lessened.

Of course, all of this is moot if we continue to eat a diet rich in saturated fats, refined carbohydrates and poor quality protein. If that were the case, all the glycine in the world would go for naught (there is evidence that excessive glycine may increase uric acid).

Now I won't go into each in detail, but I will make a couple of points you might find interesting.

Numerous studies over the years have shown what I consider a remarkable correlation that is pretty conclusive and that is that no one with multiple sclerosis has gout or elevated uric acid. It seems that both MS and gout are mutually exclusive diseases. This is an important point for any health care practitioner who is trying to diagnose multiple sclerosis which can be quite tricky. Because of this finding, some treatments for the disease have revolved around the raising of uric acid levels in MS patients.[93] The viewpoint, as Sotgiu et al had in their 2002 paper, is that depleted uric acid may be a sign of a "loss of protection against oxidative agents."[94] I couldn't be more in agreement with this train of thought.

Another interesting comment I have about MS is a small study I was part of when I was working for Life Balances, Inc. in Spokane, Washington. John Kitkoski, my mentor there, had an interesting proposition to make; he wanted to see if there was a link between potato eating and MS because of the high incidence of the disease in areas where the tuber was grown. It seemed strange at first but I learned to rarely doubt John when he made comments like this one.

Off to the library I went (no Internet searches back then) to do some epidemiological work and lo and behold MS seemed to follow a trail where whenever potatoes were introduced, MS soon followed. We then did a 10 person study where we tracked the severity and exacerbation/remission periods correlated to their ingestion of potatoes along with nutrient intake. Not surprisingly, there was a very close correlation with the quantity and frequency of eating potatoes and the exacerbation/remission periods. The more potatoes eaten, the worse the exacerbation periods and the shorter the remission periods. No claims here, just an interesting fact that should be looked at and if I had the disease, I would avoid potatoes and see what happened.

What's All the Fuss Over LDLs?

Now I will get into an area that should cause a lot of controversy, LDL and heart disease. To me it is a deceptive medical issue that has received a great deal of press and made lots of companies hundreds of billions (yes billions) of dollars. I'm not singling out the pharmaceutical industry here either as many nutritional supplement and herbal remedy purveyors are involved in this as well. If there were ever a lie wrapped up in a series of falsehoods, poured into a jar of half-truths and bundled up in a sham it is LDL and heart disease. The con game of lowering LDL to prevent heart disease is an exhibition of a three card Monte game done on the grandest scale in human history. A beautifully written book which covers this subject is *Overdo$ed America* by Dr. John Abramson.[95] It is a book everyone should have on their shelf and read cover to cover.

To understand why I've said what I did, we need to go back to an important concept in order to frame my argument. It is also somewhat controversial but it is crucial to understand and it is the concept of evolution.

Now this is not the place to get into a moral debate about God, intelligent design theory and evolution. That is something for politicians, preachers, and philosophers to debate and for you to decide personally. The evolutionary hypothesis I need to discuss is that all forms of life evolve in some form constantly. It is something that is seen and verified by millions of biologists worldwide on a regular basis.

So what does this have to do with the price of Chianti in Italy? Everything! It is a lynch pin in the discussion.

When it comes to evolution, little happens by chance. Yeah, a meteor strike here and there, massive solar flares or massive volcanic eruptions changing the earth's temperature have dramatic effects, but it is evolution, not revolution, that drives biology. The development of a complex biochemical system to deal with infectious agents of many types was not a happenstance occurrence. The same can be said for the production of low density lipoproteins (LDL).

For anyone to say that LDL is the "bad cholesterol" is to show an abundance of ignorance, a loose use of terminology meant to explain a complex subject to weak minds or a damn good marketing ploy. My choice should be obvious as I don't think that doctors are ignorant or weak minded. They are susceptible to a marketing scheme said enough times to make everyone believe it's true.

Think about it. Our bodies don't produce LDL cholesterol in order to cause heart attacks. For an organism to purposely create a metabolic process over a long period of time with no beneficial purpose or only for a negative one is patently ludicrous. Yet, if you listen to the media and the advertising for the statin drugs, you'd think that. The mantra has become "the lower the better." Any study that even hints at that is trumpeted from on high through every media channel imaginable. Anything to the contrary is relegated to a cold case file packed far away with no chance to hit the light of day.

The truth of the day is that almost half of all the people who have a heart attack have normal blood pressure, normal cholesterol, normal blood sugar and normal triglycerides! So according to the experts, there is nothing wrong with them.

Low-density lipoproteins, which are manufactured by your liver, have a number of beneficial attributes which include:

- Transporting fatty acids to your cells as a major source of energy.
- Providing a source of raw material for the creation of hormones.
- Delivering fatty acids to the heart for energy.
- Helping scavenge toxins as they flow through the blood stream.

As you can see, there are a number of benefits to low-density lipoproteins and there may be serious implications in lowering them too much in pursuit of a single-minded goal.

One of the main jobs as I mentioned above is for LDL to float around the blood stream looking for toxins to envelope and remove. Contrary to what you've seen in the media and advertising they are not just gobs of fat looking for an arterial wall to stick to. It is my firm belief (backed up by more than a little research) that often times the reason for an increased LDL level in many people is due to environmental toxins and the body's need to rid itself of the insult.

Dr. Ufe Ravnskov, a brilliant physician based in Sweden, feels that cholesterol is vital as a mechanism involved in immune response as well as being somewhat protective against atherosclerosis.[96] Of course, with all the money to be made in selling cholesterol lowering drugs, supplements and herbs, Dr. Ravnskov isn't given much heed despite solid evidence.

Whichever side you feel comfortable being on regarding cholesterol one thing should be clear, there shouldn't be a blanket statement that fits everyone. Low cholesterol is a risk factor for a number of diseases and syndromes such as cancer, depression, and suicide, as well as putting you at a higher risk to be in an accident, as was reported in an editorial for the esteemed journal "Circulation".[97] Furthermore, there is solid evidence that in people over the age of 70, lowering cholesterol does little in the way of preventing coronary heart disease.[98]

I could go on and on but the bottom line is, the marketing far outstrips the science when it comes to cholesterol. This reminds me of a scene in the movie *Sleeper* in where Woody Allen's character wakes up years after he went in for minor surgery and he discovers a new world where they've discovered that eating lard, red meat and smoking cigars was the best way to stay healthy. While this might be a bit of an exaggeration, the idea of the lower your cholesterol level is the healthier you are should be put on the same myth pedestal as the Norse gods of old.

19. MEDICINE BY REPRESENTATION

"The whole edifice of modern medicine is like the celebrated tower of Pisa – slightly off balance."

Charles, Prince of Wales

"Injections...... are the best thing ever invented for feeding doctors."

Gabriel Garcia Márquez

"We have to ask ourselves whether medicine is to remain a humanitarian and respected profession or a new but depersonalized science in the service of prolonging life rather than diminishing human suffering."

Elisabeth Kübler-Ross

"No taxation without representation" was the battle cry of the American Revolution. This was a noble cause that helped launch the United States. Unfortunately a twisted form of "representational medicine" has taken over the noble occupation of physician.

Many of today's doctors are practicing medicine by relying on pharmaceutical representatives sent in by their companies to "educate" the physician in the best ways (meaning most profitable for the company) to use their arsenal of drugs. I am sure that many of you have arrived at your doctor's office with a full waiting room not of fellow patients, but of well groomed, well dressed young pharmaceutical reps, enthusiastically filling up the little brochure containers with the "latest" information about the hot new drug or the tried and true med.

These reps go into the doctor's office and pitch the company line which is basically that their drug is great for the condition the FDA approved of due to good scientific research. They further go on to tout other, unapproved occasions that the drug should be prescribed based on "internal research" or from information gathered when they talked to other physicians on their route. These reps also talk about dinners, or gatherings in posh locations around the country where the doctor can come and find out the latest research on drug A or B. Drug companies spend billions not just millions on this and other marketing schemes.

Add to this mix, the patient coming into the office demanding a drug they saw on television promising them the ability to skip through fields of grass while gazing lovingly (and lustfully) at their wife in a happy mood if only they took this or that drug. The patient is typically tired, cranky, unable or uninterested in sex and has been depressed (or at least a little sad once in a while) and they want something to help them through the day. Of course, their excessive drinking, stressful lifestyle, and poor dietary habits have nothing to do with it or if it did it is just too much of a bother to resolve. Come on doc, give me a prescription for Clariviagranexiza™ and let me go to back to my life and be content. If you don't, Doc Holliday down the street will do it and you don't want to lose my business right?

Before the doctor gives the patient the prescription they will make an attempt to lecture them on ways of being healthier. Lose weight, cut back on the booze and quit smoking. Good advice, but with today's managed care, HMOs, and revolving door physicians offices, there is not much time to really get into a meaningful and personalized discussion.

After a while the practitioners see the patients get heavier, more stressed and less willing to change their habits so they decide that giving them the Clariviagranexizac™ will at least make their patient happy and the rep did say that it will also make athlete's foot go away and in some men, make their hair grow back on their heads. You may think this is a humorous representation of what is going on in medicine but it is not. This is medicine today.

A recent study published in the esteemed Journal of the American Medical Association (JAMA), proved that advertising was highly involved in the decision making of physicians on whether to put their patients on meds or not. The study reviewed evidence from 298 scripted visits to 152 physician's offices, between 2003 and 2004, not surprisingly they found that doctors were most likely to write prescriptions when the antidepressant Paxil® was requested.[99] This was because patients were being bombarded with advertising about this particular drug and they were convinced that they needed a prescription for it.

Physicians prescribed drugs in 53 percent of cases, with 27 percent of those for Paxil®. When patients made a more general request, however, they walked away with drugs even more often: 76 percent of the time. "We were a bit startled to see the rather high levels of prescribing for patients who made requests for medication in the adjustment disorder condition, because clinical evidence suggests that the benefits of such medication in that situation are really quite minimal," Richard Kravitz the chief investigator of the study said.

York University associate professor Joel Lexchin interviewed on Canadian television pointed out that the study bought out some of the risks associated with drug advertising.[100]

"One of the major risks is that most of the drugs that get this kind of direct consumer advertising are new products," Dr Lexchin continued to say "And new products are ones that we don't know a lot about their safety on."

In the United States alone, the pharmaceutical industry spends over $3 billion dollars a year advertising their drugs, the majority of which is targeted to the consumer, not the doctor. When I saw my first Claritin® commercial, and I was told that I could get "Claritin® Clear" I didn't know whether it was a drug to help with constipation, mental acuity or congestion. Imagine the confusion of the general public when seeing this constant bombardment of "new drug" discoveries.

Don't thinks it's a problem? Dr. Lexchin went on to warn the viewers of his interview "... you end up with problems we saw with Vioxx -- where lots of people got it inappropriately. In the United States, it's estimated to have caused between 80- and 100,000 excess cases of heart disease." Let's think about those numbers. Coldly, you can think that the treatment of those cases that should not have happened average $50,000 each (very, very conservative estimate). The additional cost to our health care system from the Vioxx debacle alone is then $5 billion dollars. This is one drug alone. There are many more.

Let's look at the drug Neurontin®. It is used in the treatment of epilepsy with a generic name of gabapentin. In 2003, over 10 million people had taken it, often times for things not related to epilepsy, such as pain. Guess what? The FDA never approved of its use for anything other than for the treatment of epilepsy.

Here is a disturbing fact about Neurontin®, the drug's prescribing information (the tiny type insert included with your prescriptions) includes a mention of "suicide gesture" as a rare side effect. A spokesman for Pfizer, the maker of the drug, said adverse event reports compiled over more than a decade "show no link between Neurontin and suicidal thoughts or behavior." Unfortunately (a word that sadly gets used often in this book), that may not be the case.

The FDA and other regulatory groups around the world are looking into the correlation between an increased risk of suicide and taking this "wonder drug". What is a human life worth here? It is also a personal issue for me because as you may recall from earlier in the book, Tasya, my dear child, has had a number of recurring emotional issues, like suicidal talk, that are most likely due to her anti-epileptic drugs (AEDs).

With Neurontin® there is more to it. They were ordered to pay over $430 million to settle both criminal and civil charges relating to improper promotion of the drug. If you think that is a lot of money, think again. The 2005 estimate of profit for Pfizer, Inc, the present owner of Warner-Lambert, is over $8 billion. The penalties laid down on them represent only 5% of their annual profits. Expressed over the past 5 years, and estimating a mere $5 billion of annual profits, that results in the equivalent of a Happy Meal at McDonald's for the corporate giant. Do you see something wrong here?

The following is a quote from the "FDA Consumer" magazine of July/August 2004.

> *Pharmaceutical manufacturer Warner-Lambert has agreed to plead guilty and pay more than $430 million to resolve criminal charges and civil liabilities in connection with its Parke-Davis division's illegal and fraudulent promotion of unapproved uses for the drug Neurontin (gabapentin). The drug was approved by the Food and Drug Administration in December 1993 solely for use with other drugs to control seizures in people with epilepsy.*
>
> *Under the provisions of the Federal Food, Drug, and Cosmetic Act, a company must specify the intended uses of a product in its new drug application to the FDA. Once approved, the drug may not be marketed or promoted for so-called "off-label" uses--any use not specified in an application and approved by the FDA.*
>
> *Warner-Lambert's strategic marketing plans, as well as other evidence, show that Neurontin was aggressively marketed to treat a wide array of ailments for which the drug was not approved, according to a recent press statement from the U.S. Department of Justice. The company promoted Neurontin for the treatment of:*
>
> * *bipolar mental disorder*
> * *various pain disorders*
> * *amyotrophic lateral sclerosis (ALS), commonly referred to as Lou Gehrig's disease*
> * *attention-deficit disorder*
> * *migraine*
> * *drug and alcohol withdrawal seizures*
> * *restless leg syndrome*
>
> *The company also promoted the drug as a first-line monotherapy treatment for epilepsy--using Neurontin alone, rather than in addition to another drug.*

Warner-Lambert promoted Neurontin even when scientific studies had shown it was not effective. For example, the company promoted Neurontin as effective for use as the sole drug for epileptic seizures, even after sole use had been specifically rejected by the FDA. Similarly, the pharmaceutical company falsely promoted Neurontin as effective for treating bipolar disorder, even when a scientific study demonstrated that a placebo worked as well or better than the drug.

"This illegal and fraudulent promotion scheme corrupted the information process relied upon by doctors in their medical decision-making, thereby putting patients at risk," says U.S. Attorney Michael Sullivan. "This scheme deprived federally-funded Medicaid programs across the country of the informed, impartial judgment of medical professionals--judgment on which the program relies to allocate scarce financial resources to provide necessary and appropriate care to the poor. The pharmaceutical industry will not be allowed to profit from such conduct nor subject the poor, the elderly, and other persons insured by state and federal health care programs to experimental drug uses which have not been determined to be safe and effective."

As a consequence of the unlawful promotion scheme, patients who received the drug for unapproved and unproven uses had no assurance that their doctors were exercising their independent and fully informed medical judgment or whether the doctor was instead influenced by misleading statements or inducements from Warner-Lambert. Potential problems that can arise from off-label use without the benefit of careful FDA oversight include the occurrence of unforeseen problems because the drug was not studied in the type of patient it is being used for off-label, and the appropriate dosage and course of treatment have not been established.

Warner-Lambert used a number of tactics to achieve its marketing goals, including encouraging sales representatives to provide one-on-one sales pitches to physicians about off-label uses of Neurontin without prior inquiry by doctors. The company's agents also made false or misleading statements to health care professionals regarding Neurontin's efficacy and whether it had been approved by the FDA for the off-label uses. Warner-Lambert also used "medical liaisons," who represented themselves (often falsely) as scientific experts in a particular disease, to promote off-label uses for Neurontin.

Warner-Lambert paid doctors to attend so-called "consultants' meetings" in which physicians received a fee for attending expensive dinners or conferences during which presentations about off-label uses of Neurontin were made. These events included lavish weekends and trips to Florida, the 1996 Atlanta Olympics, and Hawaii. There was little or no significant consulting provided by the physicians.

The pharmaceutical company implemented numerous teleconferences in which physicians were recruited by sales representatives to call into a prearranged number where they would listen to a doctor or Warner-Lambert employee speak about off-label use of Neurontin. The company also sponsored purportedly "independent medical education" events on off-label Neurontin uses with extensive input from Warner-Lambert regarding topics, speakers, content, and participants.

Warner-Lambert misled the medical community beforehand about the content, as well as the lack of independence from the company's influence, of many of these educational events. In at least one instance, when unfavorable remarks were proposed by a speaker, Warner-Lambert offset the negative impact by "planting" people in the audience to ask questions highlighting the benefits of the drug.

Warner-Lambert paid physicians to allow a sales representative to accompany the physician while he or she saw patients, with the representative offering advice regarding the patient's treatment that was biased toward the use of Neurontin.

These tactics were part of a widespread, coordinated national effort to implement an off-label marketing plan. At the same time, Warner-Lambert decided not to seek FDA approval for any of the new uses because it was concerned that approval for any of the non-epilepsy uses would allow generic competitors of Neurontin to compete with a "son of Neurontin" drug that Warner-Lambert hoped to have approved by the FDA for both epilepsy and non-epilepsy uses.

Neurontin was put on the market in February of 1994. From mid-1995 to at least 2001, the growth of off-label sales was tremendous. While not all of these sales were the consequence of Warner-Lambert's illegal marketing, the marketing scheme was very successful in increasing Neurontin prescriptions for unapproved uses.

The investigation began in the District of Massachusetts when a former medical liaison for Warner-Lambert, David Franklin, M.D., filed suit on behalf of the U.S. government. Private individuals are allowed to file whistleblower suits under the federal False Claims Act to bring the United States information about wrongdoing. If the United States is successful in resolving or litigating the whistleblower's claims, the whistleblower may share part of the recovery. As a part of the resolution, Franklin will receive about $24.6 million of the civil recovery.

The Federal Bureau of Investigation, the Department of Veterans Affairs' Office of Criminal Investigations, the FDA's Office of Criminal Investigations, and the Office of Inspector General for the Department of Health and Human Services conducted the investigation.

Terms of the agreement include:

- *Warner-Lambert has agreed to plead guilty to two counts of violating the Federal Food, Drug, and Cosmetic Act with regard to its misbranding of Neurontin by failing to provide adequate directions for use and by introduction into interstate commerce of an unapproved new drug. Warner-Lambert has, as punishment for these offenses, agreed to pay a $240 million criminal fine, the second-largest criminal fine ever imposed in a health care fraud prosecution.*
- *Warner-Lambert has agreed to settle its federal civil False Claims Act liabilities and to pay the United States $83.6 million, plus interest, in civil damages for losses suffered by the federal portion of the Medicaid program as a result of Warner-Lambert's fraudulent drug promotion and marketing misconduct.*
- *Warner-Lambert has agreed to settle its civil liabilities to the 50 states and the District of Columbia in an amount of $38 million, plus interest, for harm caused to consumers and to fund a remediation program to address the effects of Warner-Lambert's improper marketing scheme.*
- *Pfizer Inc., Warner-Lambert's parent company, has agreed to comply with the terms of a corporate compliance program, which will ensure that the changes Pfizer Inc. made after acquiring Warner-Lambert in June 2000 are effective in training and supervising its marketing and sales staff.*

If after reading this you do not get angry or at least frightened, something is very wrong. Not only that but trusted institutions such as Emory University Hospital still tout Neurontin® on their website for some of the unapproved conditions. To top it off they make no mention of the increased risk of suicide from the use of gabapentin. Want to know a possible reason, just look into who is funding their research.

I have been approached by many who claim that this is an example of the grand conspiracy that the major pharmaceutical companies are participating in. I shrug my shoulders and beg to disagree. Greed makes people do things that often times resemble collusionary behavior. It is a product of our economic system. To steal a quote from Lord Acton and give it the Schauss Twist, "A little greed corrupts a little bit, absolute greed corrupts absolutely."

The drive of CEOs to continue increasing profits in today's economy is forcing what may be good people to become so engrossed with absolute greed and the pressure to keep stock prices up that they never see the corruption they become enveloped with.

Having said all of that you might get the idea that I am radically opposed to drugs and pharmaceuticals. Au contraire. Don't get me wrong, I am not anti-pharmaceutical, far from it. Discoveries in the field of pharmaceutical drugs have been life saving and life improving for millions of people worldwide. In the book, *"Powerful Medicines: The Benefits, Risks, and Costs of Prescription Drugs"* by Dr. Jerry Avorn,[101] we see the triumphs and travesties of how we use drugs in America.

My beef is with the ill-advised, often times non-scientific and medically unnecessary use of these powerful chemicals. The way medicine is being run today is nothing more than marketing products to customers. What happened to treating a patient, finding out what caused the disease and treating that instead of trying to only treat the symptoms?

Treatment of disease in today's model is becoming nothing more than cosmetic medicine. That is to say that most of the way medicine deals with health related issues is to cover up the problem much like makeup covers up an ugly blemish on your face, with one very different side effect. With makeup, you have minor side effects from its use, with drugs you may have serious ones.

In the case of depression, today's model is to prescribe Paxil®, Prozac® or some other powerful medication. Ever hear of a Paxil®

deficiency? Nope, neither have I. Have amino acid deficiencies like tyrosine or tryptophan been linked to depression? You bet they have. Adding those two in deficient patients has yielded remarkable results as well, but that is something I will cover in the section on amino acids. Why do we constantly run to the extreme remedy like a drug without trying to uncover causative factors like nutrient or amino acid deficiencies?

One interesting side note here on depression is the use of the herb St. John's Wort. If you believe the media, it was a terrible failure in its ability to help people with moderate to severe depression. It was big news carried by all the major media outlets which get a majority of the advertising dollars spread around by the pharmaceutical industry. What the reporters covering the story mysteriously failed to mention was that the placebo affect that St. John's Wort was compared to was strangely lower than any other study previously done compared to drugs.[102] Also, the study showed that it was helpful in some moderate depression but most naturopaths would agree that its use is mostly for minor depression. In a subsequent study the herb was actually found to do quite well in moderate cases of depression.

Another discussion about the pharmaceutical industry is how they manipulate patent laws and create new "wonder drugs" which really aren't that new after all. A case in point is the "purple pill" Nexium®. This drug is really only supposed to be used in severe cases of heartburn where esophageal erosion has occurred but the numbers here are relatively small. It only represents about 10% of severe heartburn patients; hardly enough to justify its release financially, especially since there was already an effective drug on the market made by the same manufacturer, AstraZeneca, known as Prilosec OTC® (marketed by partner Procter and Gamble). So why release it at all? Are you not competing with yourself? That makes no sense until you understand the patent issue and drugs.

Patents are protection to the industry for their hard work in researching novel drugs. They are supposed to let the companies market the drug they developed, without any competition so they can profit from it. No problem here. The problem I have is that Nexium® and Prilosec® are essentially the same product with a slight difference that allows Nexium® to become patented, thus allowing AstraZeneca to reap the rewards for a new drug development. Prilosec, was no longer protected under patent so generic competitors could come into the market. It also got approved by the FDA for over the counter status allowing it to be purchased without a prescription. Which one of the two drugs do you think has a higher profit margin? Yup, it is definitely Nexium®.

The bottom line though would be if Nexium® is substantially better than Prilosec® then this discussion is moot. Problem is, it is not substantially better, just a little bit. The same is true for so many of the drugs on the market today. In reality, as an example, to get a new anti-epileptic drug approved, you only have to show a 50% improvement in seizure control in 50% of the patients with a little decrease in side-effects to be approved by the FDA. The incentive is to constantly make more and more of the New Improved Tide® instead of making breakthroughs because it is easier and cheaper. Profit over everything seemingly is the mantra of the pharmaceutical industry.

One last tidbit of information before we move off of this topic is the scale of the profits the pharmaceutical industry has reaped. In the books *"The Truth About the Drug Companies"* by Dr. Marcia Angell[103] and *"The $800 Million Pill: The Truth Behind the Cost of Drugs"* by Merrill Goozner,[104] they show how incredible the numbers are. They also lay waste to the claims by the industry on how expensive it is to do the research to make all of these supposed breakthroughs (Viagra®, Cialis® and Levitra® are all life saving eh?). To put it mildly, it's a scam of the highest proportions.

The top twenty pharmaceutical companies made more profits in the past twenty years than the combined profits of the other 480 Fortune 500 companies did over the same period. The industries claim that there is inherent risk in developing a drug because with all their research, the drug may not be approved, thus wasting all that money. That is not a bad argument if the risk/reward ratio was not so out of whack. Unfortunately (there is that word again), the numbers do not lie. This industry is making more money with less risk than any other one in the world. Period.

Here is a final list of the kind of numbers we are talking about; something to take home with you.

Top 20 Pharmaceutical Companies based on 2002 revenues which totals over $246 billion

1. Pfizer $28,288
2. GlaxoSmithKline $27,060
3. Merck $20,130
4. AstraZeneca $17,841
5. J&J $17,151
6. Aventis $16,639
7. Bristol-Myers Squibb $14,705
8. Novartis $13,547
9. Pharmacia $12,037
10. Wyeth $10,899
11. Lilly $10,385
12. Abbott $9,700
13. Roche $9,355
14. Schering-Plough $8,745
15. Takeda $7,031
16. Sanofi $7,045
17. Boehringer-Ingelheim $5,369
18. Bayer $4,509
19. Schering AG $3,074
20. Sankyo $2,845

2002 R&D Expenditures which totals $45,587,000,000 or 19% of the total revenues

1. Pfizer $5,176
2. GlaxoSmithKline $4,108
3. J&J $3,957
4. AstraZeneca $3,069
5. Aventis $3,235
6. Novartis $2,799
7. Roche $2,746
8. Merck $2,677
9. Bristol-Myers Squibb $2,218
10. Pharmacia $2,359
11. Wyeth $2,080
12. Lilly $2,149

13. Abbott $1,562
14. Schering-Plough $1,425
15. Boehringer-Ingelheim $1,304
16. Sanofi $1,152
17. Takeda $1,020
18. Bayer $1,014
19. Schering AG $896
20. Sankyo $641

Oh and not all R&D expenditures are devoted to pharmaceuticals. Darn, I'm in the wrong business. I should have been a pharmaceutical company when I grew up

One other issue I'd like to bring up that will be a little controversial to some in the alternative health world and that is regarding a conspiracy by the pharmaceutical industry to squash nutritional supplements because they are taking money away from "big pharma." While I have no doubt that there are a number of disinformationists working within the industry and that there are a number of individuals who are very anti-supplements, I think we need to be very clear that these companies are probably not overly concerned about the amount of money supplements are taking away from them.

Let's put the numbers into perspective. As you saw with the list of revenues from the top 20 pharmaceutical companies, the total income exceeded $246 billion in 2002. The total revenues generated from all natural product including cosmetics, foods, and supplements in the U.S. in 2003 was $20.5 billion.[105] Estimates suggest that the total of supplement sales at the high end represents 40% of this total or about $8.2 billion. This comes out to around 3% of the gross sales of the pharmaceutical giants and I can tell you honestly that the profit margins are a lot less for the supplement companies than for big pharma.

What we need is legislation to reverse the marketing power of the pharmaceutical industry so we can lower the cost of medicine and reduce the number of errors made from the gross abuse of drugs.

20. The Three Blind Monkey Theory: How hucksters can be made to look like geniuses

"Man's mind is so formed that it is far more susceptible to falsehood than to truth."

Desiderius Erasmus

"Every man is a potential genius until he does something."

Sir Herbert Beerbohm Tree

"A deception that elevates us is dearer than a host of low truths."

Marina Tsvetaeva

Lest you think I am strictly anti-pharmaceutical and think that "if it's natural, it must be safe," read this chapter and understand that both sides of the aisle have problems.

Being involved in the world of alternative medicine on and off for the past 20+ years has given me an insight into a world filled with some of the most caring, helpful and genuine people you could ever hope to meet. It has also shown me the dark underbelly of humankind which could make anyone jaded and suspicious about everyone. Thankfully, I was able to see through those types of people and focus more on the positives than the negatives. Still, I think it is necessary to arm the reader with tools to avoid falling into the quack trap.

Imagine you have a dreaded incurable disease and have tried every known therapy with a continuingly worsening prognosis. Then you hear about an alternative treatment known as the Watermelon and raw Meat Diet that requires you to only eat watermelons, their seeds and raw meats, but considering you have little hope otherwise, you are going to try it out despite the fact that it logically makes no sense. Strangely enough, it seems to be working, as you slowly get better. You go back to the doctor and he seems astounded, your terminal disease has gone away and you are as good as gold. What you fail to realize is that the treatments that you were using, perhaps chemotherapy, radiation or a rational nutritional program, all of whom you recently discontinued, had kicked in and worked despite the odds.

You now make it your mission to tell the world that the Watermelon and Meat Diet (also known as the WMD) saved your life and is the greatest thing since sliced Gouda cheese. Also, if you dare criticize the WMD I will accuse you of being anti-health, anti-American, or worse, an evil person. Criticize the WMD and you will be vilified, cursed and at times threatened. Don't think this happens? It happens all the time and it is at the core of many of the snake oil products being sold today.

A while back on a Yahoo newsgroup, I got into a tiff with a person who was hawking a multi-level vitamin supplement. At first glance it seemed perfectly fine but when he proudly proclaimed that there were 90+ minerals in his "life-saving" product, I became suspicious as humans do not need that many and it most likely included toxic heavy metals. When I began to research the product, lo and behold, in the ingredients list, there were mercury, cadmium, arsenic, aluminum and lead. When I questioned him about this and pointed out that these were unwanted toxins, he went after me viciously.

The first shot he fired was that I did not know what I was talking about and that the "experts" who ran the company were brilliant doctors and scientists. And he and his family were getting better so my claims about toxicity were pointless. When that didn't work the attacks became stranger.

After contacting his superior in the multi-level marketing scheme, they told him that what I did not realize is that the elements were "organic" so this somehow makes them safer. When I replied with a series of studies that pointed out that with some of the metals, organic forms were far more toxic that the non-organic forms,[106] he began to boil over with his anger and the following line was posted, truly amazing me:

"You show your ignorance Mark loud and clear because if you were halfway intelligent you would understand that God put those organic minerals on our planet for our use and He would not do that unless it were good for you. So go away to your Godless world."

HUH????

To say I was stunned by this line of logic is the understatement of the year. I guess deadly toxic mushrooms were placed on this earth for good reasons for our consumption? This of course is an extreme example of hucksterism but variations of this are not that uncommon. Here is another example of the problems with the nutritional supplement world.

I was sitting with a friend at a chiropractic relicensing conference and we noticed that two men were arguing rather vociferously. As we leaned forward to hear what the argument was all about my friend began to grin and chuckle. The two men, who we were thinking might be getting into a physical fight if things do not de-escalate, were accusing each other of having inferior forms of CoEnzyme Q10, and were ripping people off. My friend leans over to me and whispers, "Guess what Mark? I manufacture both of their CoQ10s and as a matter of fact, they are made at the same time, same batch and there is no difference between the two except the guy on the right charges 50% more for his with a fancier label and nicer marketing package."

There are a number of examples where vitamin manufacturers are selling the same product for wildly different prices with some making outrageous claims. So what is a consumer to do? You have to find someone to trust who can help you find out what is real and what is not. This is part of what I did at Carbon Based Corporation. I tried to help the health care practitioner, and at times, individuals find out what is real and what is not.

I do not want the reader to think that this is a rampant problem and that you need to be suspicious of all the supplement companies. There are a large number of real honest and ethically run companies you can find in the resource section of this book. A caveat, an omission of a company's name does not mean they are bad or unethical nor do I claim to know every single supplement company that exists. I cannot name everyone who is doing a good job although I wish I could. The list is just those I know of and have confidence in. If you are a company I omitted, please contact me and we can talk and you may get included in my next edition.

The problem of hucksterism does not end with supplement companies; there are testing laboratories and so-called "experts" in the field on health that are the worst offenders and are the worst abusers of the "Three Blind Monkey Theory" also known as the TBMT.

So what is this TBMT??? And how does it pertain to health and hucksters.

Imagine putting three blind monkeys into a room with darts. The walls are covered with nutritional supplement recommendations. The monkeys are trained to throw the darts against the wall and when their handlers come back in the room, they gather the information and produce a "computerized report" that takes the "monkeys" work and recommends it to the patient of the doctor they are working with. They do this under the guise of a lab test, questionnaire or some advanced computerized system.

The patient is now sent on their way with a bag full of nutrients not really understanding why but feeling confident that this "scientific" method was state-of-the-art and the best that money could buy.

Some people have worked very hard to put together systems that use the TBMT theory with good intentions. Some, unfortunately with less than honorable intentions. But Mark, how can they stay in business, won't people catch on?

Not necessarily and here is the reason why.

The monkeys, after throwing their darts came up with the following nutritional supplement and herbal recommendations: Vitamin **B**1, Oil of **O**regano, **M**agnesium, Vitamin **B**6, **S**elenium, Vitamin **A**, **W**atercress extract, Ashwaganda and Yohimbine (The new product is named **BOMBS AWAY**). The marketing gurus thought that focusing on males between the ages of 40-60 would make the most sense. With this new product combination they could get a positive response rate approaching forty percent!!!

Pretty impressive you might say? I would be appalled because I look at this glass as not being forty percent full but being sixty percent empty. Further review reveals that forty percent of the people who took **BOMBS AWAY** saw no difference in their health and twenty percent got worse. Sixty percent of the people threw money out the window and got no significant benefits from this relatively expensive product.

Remember the first example with the WMD diet plan? The person who got benefits from the diet will tell the world about their positive experience even though it might have nothing to do with their recovery at all. Say you had 5000 people try the BOMBS AWAY product at $100 per bottle and 40% got positive results and re-ordered the product once. If your cost was $10 for each bottle of the product here is what it would look like:

1. $100 times 5,000 orders equals $500,000
2. 40% first time reorder rate equals 2,000 reorders times $100 equals $200,000
3. 40% second time reorder rate (from #2) equals 800 reorders times $100 equals $80,000
4. 40% third order rate time 800 equals 320 orders which equals $32,000.
5. The number of orders comes out to 8,200 orders or $820,000
6. The cost of the orders is 8,200 times $10 or $82,000
7. The gross profit is $820,000 minus $82,000 or $738,000!!!

Not bad for a few months work, right? Pretty good for a sixty percent failure rate as well! To the remaining 320 people from the original 5,000 you have a loyal marketing force, convinced that this product saved them. Mark, hey don't you see that you've helped those 320 people get better and isn't that the bottom line?

NO IT ISN'T.

If you use the concept of biochemical individuality, you can do a whole lot better and not waste the money of the 93.6% of the people who received no long term benefits from the product (5000[total buys]-320[those who received long term benefits]/5000=93.6%.). The three blind monkeys can make a killing every year for their handlers if they can replicate this a few times.

Abe Lincoln, when posed the following question, made a profound statement as he was known to do:

Mr. Lincoln, if you call a horse's tail a leg, how many legs does the horse have? "Four" Mr. Lincoln replied, "Calling a horse's tail a leg does not make it one."

In the world of lab testing there are two examples that you need to be aware of.

There is a lab which claims that their tests indicate that autistic kids have major yeast infections which are unique to these children. No problem here (although I disagree with the premise). The doctors who get these results decide to treat their patients with Diflucan (an anti-fungal drug). Sixty percent of the kids show dramatic improvement with the treatment and the lab touts the results as proving their theory.

Problem is the labs results that indicated a yeast infection are not scientifically valid. A matter of fact, the results have only minor correlations with yeast. So what is really happening here?

In the world of toxicity, there are two phases of detoxification, I and II. In phase I, the toxin is oxidized (although not always) to create an intermediary chemical which is commonly more toxic than the original toxin.[107] These intermediaries can be quite neurotoxic, especially to autistic children. These children also have impaired phase II detox capacities which allow these intermediaries more time to do damage both direct and indirect.

What some of the anti-fungal drugs do is potentially down-regulate (slow down) phase I detoxification. If we slow down phase I, we slow down the production of the neurotoxic intermediaries and thereby allow to impaired phase II to keep up.

The kids get better!!!

Does it have anything to do with yeast? Maybe and maybe not. Does it help the child? For the short term yes. Long term? Not so sure about that. But it makes the lab look darn good because the parents of the kids who are desperate for any improvement are overjoyed. Is the horse's tail a leg?

While these children are alleviating the short term intermediary toxic insult, they do a number of things that improve phase II (increasing amino acid competency) which removes more toxins, they get off the Diflucan and they recover from autism. So what's wrong with that?

Lots.

Using drugs like Diflucan and Nystatin (another anti-fungal) can lead to drug resistant yeast to proliferate (the bugs can evolve quite easily) which can negatively impact the individual later on in life. Antibiotic resistance is a major problem in today's health care world.

To use anti-fungals irresponsibly is bad medicine and is not only bad for the individual but the public as a whole. It is helping to create genetically modified species of yeast to gain a short term benefit, which borders on malpractice. Don't get depressed though. There is a better way!!!

The first thing to do is to lower the toxic load and balance the phase I / phase II detox pathways. One way is to assess the pathway using a simple urine test from a reputable lab (such as MetaMetrix) which can determine both phases' capacities. Then, by adjusting the ratios of phase I and II, you can improve efficiency which will prevent creating the toxic intermediary chemicals which can cause neurological and other health issues. This will help issues relating to long-term health.

By the way, with autistic children, their health concerns do not begin and end with autistic spectrum disorder (ASD). There are many other issues that need to be dealt with and treatments have to be created that will not cause additional harm. We need to look at the bigger picture here.

Another example of the TBMT is from another laboratory interpretive reporting company who was making the outrageous claim that people in the US are higher in Omega 3 fatty acids that Omega 6s. You may be smirking since the world's research contradicts this claim but they made the claim nonetheless. In this case I think they were asking if the horse's rear end was a leg.

Here is why there is a problem with their testing protocol:

A highly touted test by some in the alternative health field is the red cell membrane fatty acid test. There are two differing methods of reporting results available. One reports the actual amount/concentration of each element in the test, while the other method reports the relative percentage of the elements.

One unfortunately common example of this misinterpretation is when it is falsely stated that children with autism (as well as the general population) have higher omega 3 fatty acids than omega 6 Fatty Acids. This is in direct contradiction to published research. It is the purpose of this part of the book is to explain why such results cannot be trusted to make any health-related assessment, and how doing so can cause severe problems.

According to the book "Laboratory Evaluations in Molecular Medicine" by Drs. Bralley and Lord, one of the most profound problems with using percentage calculations is the effect abundant fatty acids have on the less abundant ones.[108]

A simple example, taken from their highly recommended book, clearly illustrates this problem:

	Case A		Case B
		Concentration	
Total FA	2000		4000
Palmitic	1000		2000
GLA	1 low		1 low
		Percentage	
Palmitic	50%		50%
GLA	.05% normal		.025% low

As you can see, the concentration of gamma linolenic acid (GLA) is low, but due to the use of the percentage assessment method, it is normal in Case A. This of course would be an incorrect statement and could lead to improper supplementation recommendations.

Here is a visualization that might better explain this phenomenon. Say you have a jar filled with layers of different colored marbles (4000 marbles total). 50% of these marbles are red (2000) and 10% are yellow (400). If we remove 500 of the red marbles they drop to 42.86% of the total (now 3500 marbles) the yellow marbles now become 11.43% of the total (400/3500) with no additional yellow marbles added. If the "reference range" of yellow marbles is 10.5 to 11.5, they would have gone from being deficient (10%) to being on the high side of normal (11.43%) without any change in concentration.

Another problem arises if the total concentration of all fatty acids is below normal, which is commonplace with ASD children. Using a percentage assessment method with low total concentration could lead to exaggerated and flawed reporting of imbalances. This would not be seen when using the proper concentration-assessment method of laboratory reporting. Here is an example of this problem:

Total content of RBC fatty acids of individual #1 is 1400 (considered low)

Total content of RBC fatty acids of individual #2 is 2400 (considered normal)

Both have a percentage of arachidonic acid (AA, a pro-inflammatory omega 6 fatty acid) of 12%, with a reference range of 13% - 16%.

The concentration of AA in the red blood cells of individual #1 would be 168.

The concentration of AA in the red blood cells of individual #2 would be 288.

According to the percentage assessment method, both would be deficient in arachidonic acid, but according to the concentration method, there is a sizeable difference between the two. It is because of this mathematical problem that false deficiencies as well as false excesses often arise.

To further compound the problem, others use the "% Status" calculations originally developed by myself back in 1985. This calculation uses a simple, yet elegant mathematical formula to allow for the relative comparison of laboratory test results having different reference ranges, as well as different units of measure.

In a nutshell, if the reference range of an element such as sodium were 135 to 148 mE/q, a 0% deviation would be the mid-point 141.5. A reading of 135 would be -50% and a result of 148 would be +50%. Using this method, one could compare the relative difference between sodium of 143 (+11.54%) and a lymphocyte of 44 (+43.75%) with a reference range of 14 to 46. When used properly, the equation allows the application of the data to a vast array of medical knowledge.

Using the percentage assessment method, both readings for arachidonic acid would be -83.33%. If we determine that the reference range for arachidonic acid is 200 – 300 using the concentration assessment model, then the first individual would be -82% (consistent with the percentage assessment model), but the second would be a positive 38%! Using the percentage assessment method on the second person might have wrongly determined a deficiency in arachidonic acid where actually a slight excess is evident.

Incorrect assessment can lead to potentially damaging recommendations. There is evidence that giving certain susceptible individuals omega 6 fatty acids can induce seizures. Also, arachidonic acid is a pro-inflammatory fatty acid that has been implicated in arthritis and coronary heart disease (amongst others).

The bottom line is to beware of using old, out-dated methodology to determine imbalances in your patient's or your own chemistries. The consequences could be highly detrimental and could cause dangerous side effects.

Thousands of people have spent thousands of dollars on this protocol with many having negative results, but enough people, aka TBMT advocates (6.3% probably got great results), prevail to allow them to continue in business.

Of course, my three blind monkeys are just a figment of my imagination but the reality is that many people use this theory, often times inadvertently, and believe that what they are recommending is safe and proven efficacious.

Following is one last example of the problems with health claims that belongs in this discussion. There is an MLM (multi-level marketing) who may or may not have a decent product but they brag about their studies showing that coal miners who take their product excrete more heavy metals than did the placebo controlled group. The study was constructed using a double-blind methodology which attempts to make sure that there is no bias in who gets the placebo and who does ntt. The study at first glance looked convincing. When you get deeper, it shows that it is deeply flawed.

In the study, there were 40 people on the "product" and only 10 getting a placebo. Squaring the two groups so that the numbers are similar should have been done to improve the study. Secondly, doing a study of this nature only against a placebo and not another known chelator of heavy metals is somewhat deceptive. To validate the product it is important to see if it is as good as or better than other products out there. To tout something as superior to others and yet not test it against other products borders on deception. In reality, many inexpensive trace mineral supplements will accomplish similar success rates when it comes to increasing the excretion of heavy metals at one third of the cost of the MLM product in question.

With any MLM, it is the goal of the top people to utilize the concept of the TBMT in order to sell the product and get it moving early on. As many know, it is the top line sellers who get in early and bring on others underneath them to sell, and who make the majority of the profits. All they need are some well-groomed, titled individuals who put together a flashy program with good sounding research and off they go.

All we need are more people who expose the shams for what they really are; just three blind monkeys sitting in a room throwing darts.

21. What the Model of Health Needs to Be

"People who don't know how to keep themselves healthy ought to have the decency to get themselves buried, and not waste time about it."

Henrik Ibsen

"Of all the anti-social vested interests the worst is the vested interest in ill-health."

George Bernard Shaw

"Health is a state of complete physical, mental and social well-being, and not merely the absence of disease or infirmity."

Constitution, The World Health Organization

In today's world of modern medicine, one would hope that the focus of research would be towards the cause of disease, but with the growing trends in pharmaceutical medicine, treatment of symptoms seems to be where most of the money goes. In the early days, finding out that an amoeba caused dysentery or certain bacteria and viruses caused other diseases was critical in providing treatment options such as antibiotics. Today there is an attempt to overuse this important tool to the point of creating a myopic thought process which is hindering the treatment of diseases such as epilepsy in order to create a seemingly comfortable environment for health professionals to operate.

All too often the focus on a single etiology blurs the fact that there may be multiple "bullets" being loaded into the "gun" that finally goes off resulting in the disease presenting itself. With epilepsy, the presentation obviously starts with the first seizure. Because we look for a direct cause-and-effect scenario, quite often the individual or more often the parent of the child with epilepsy is left hearing the comment: "We don't know why you or your child is epileptic, but here are some drugs that may help. If that doesn't work, or if upping the dose fails, we have a good selection of pharmaceuticals that in some combination may help you or your child, live with the disorder." This reminds me of the way we used to concoct new drinks when I was a bartender going through college. Mix some alcohols, sodas, and juices together and see what we get. If it doesn't taste good, try another combo.

If we look at epilepsy through a multi-factorial design, we have a better chance of determining proper protocols to not only allow for control of the seizure activity but in finding the many reasons that led to the onset of epileptic activity and hopefully prevent further seizures or help others avoid developing epilepsy.

My discussion will focus on this disorder for obvious reasons, but you should be able to see how the ideas I present can be correlated to a number of other disorders.

EPILEPSY

Epilepsy is diagnosed when there is recurrent seizure activity seen with altered consciousness, abnormal motor activity or sensory phenomena. Convulsive seizures are the main expression of the disorder characterized by tonic or clonic (rhythmic jerking movements of the arms and legs) jerking. It is not considered a disease though; rather it is considered a disorder of the nervous system. The word epilepsy derives from the ancient Greek word *epilepsia* which means "*to be seized by forces from without*".

STATISTICS

Approximately, 1.4 million Americans currently suffer from epilepsy, the majority being under the age of 45 but with an incidence highest amongst those over the age of 65 (4.6 per 1000 under 45 versus 6.2 per 1000 over the age of 65). Further investigation shows the incidence being slightly higher in females than males in most age groups. Also, the highest incidence per 1000 individuals is in the Midwest (7.9) versus the Northeast (4.4), South (3.7) and the West (4.6).

TRADITIONAL TREATMENT

Traditional treatment today revolves around 16 medications (table 1) that have been approved by the Food and Drug Administration. Typically monotherapy, using one drug, is the first step in treating the patient as multi-drug therapy seems to amplify the side-effects. Combinations are often used when monotherapy fails to control the seizure activity.

Table 1

Carbamazapine	Valproate	Phenytoin	Ethosuximide
Clonazepam	Phenobarbital	Primidone	Tiagabine
Lamotrigine	Gabapentin	Topiramate	Levtitacetam
Felbamate	Zonisamide	Oxcarbazapine	Fosphenytion

Each of these medications presents different risks and side effects. Women, especially those of child-bearing age, are told to be especially careful as some of the drugs can interfere with the effectiveness of birth control pills. Side effects commonly noted are fatigue, weight gain, dizziness and behavioral changes. More serious side effects can lead to liver failure, depression and psychosis.

So how does this model used by the allopathic community look? Here is how I visualize it:

A Multi Factorial Design for the Etiology of Disease
Classic Allopathic Model

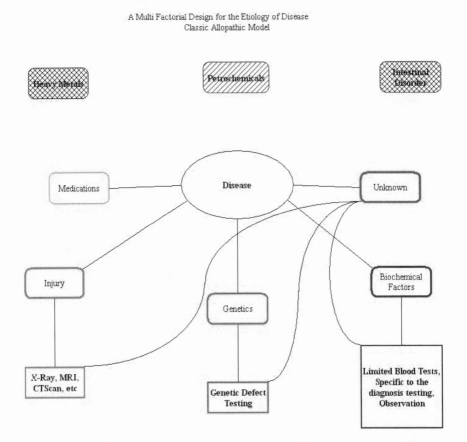

Note how the classic model has three common causations for epilepsy: injury, disease, and unknown. Over the past 10 years, genetics has become the new catch all, quickly passing unknown as a leading cause. Problem with that theory is while a good percentage of people with a certain "defective" gene may have epilepsy, many with the same bad gene do not. What is not addressed is discovering the triggers that cause the gene to express.

This theory is better described, although not thoroughly enough, by the alternative health model of disease which begins to look at disease in a multi-factorial manner:

A Multi Factorial Design for the Etiology of Disease
Traditional Alternative Approach

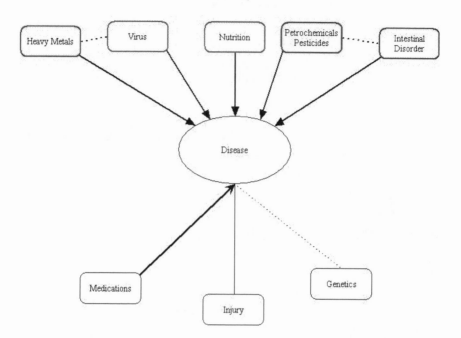

Here we see the causations being quite a bit different than in the allopathic model. Coming into play are issues like toxicity (heavy metals, petrochemicals, and pesticides), nutrition, intestinal issues, and viruses. Medications and injury play a lesser role (although still significant where applicable). Genetics takes the smallest role but that is changing as alternative health practitioners are being allured by the sexiness of a theory they really do not understand.

One of the problems I see is when you hear lecturers out on the circuit touting their "answer" to a problem. You might hear someone talking about autism saying that mercury is the only culprit or that oxalates or stealth viruses are the cause. Rarely will you hear people talking about the complexity of causation but this is where the focus must go.

With the advent of the computer age has come the ability to look at complex issues and devise treatment protocols that are much more sophisticated than what is being used today. This is why I developed the Carbon Based Method. My first two patents were on the use of multi-factorial designs in determining disease patterns, drug interactions, and organ systems reviews as well as nutritionally individualized programs based on the results of laboratory tests.

In the April 20th 2006 issue of *Nature* magazine, Clayton et al, wrote an article entitled, *Pharmaco-metabonomic phenotyping and personalized drug treatment*.[109] This landmark study shows that our biochemical individuality is crucial in being able to administer drugs and to affect other health related issues.

The authors state that drugs affect laboratory animals with similar genetics differently based upon "variation in metabolic phenotype, which is influenced not only by genotype but also by environmental factors such as nutritional status, the gut microbiota, age, disease and the co- or ore-administration of other drugs." Of course, being funded by Pfizer, they focus myopically at drug interventions (although in the last line they do mention dietary challenges) but since beginning my work in 1985 I believed that this form of "metabonomic phenotyping" was the wave of the future over even genetics, which the authors admit that "it seems unlikely that personalized drug therapy will be enabled for a wide range of major diseases using genomic knowledge alone." They used many of the same markers as those found in Urinary Organic Acid testing which I recommend regularly.

The authors also comment that "metabolite profiling of fluids other than urine, such as blood and fecal extracts, should also provide additional information", which I find interesting as this is exactly what Carbon Based Corporation had been doing for years. My company was the first one to combine test results from blood, urine, and fecal testing and we are still the only ones to do that from multiple labs. Clayton et al further states that "...we envisage that similar methodology could also be applied to predicting individual responses to broader medical, dietary, microbiological or physiological challenges." Dr. Clayton and his group do not need to look to the future as Carbon Based Corporation/Crayhon Research has already been doing this for over 12 years.

The idea of metabonomics (the variation of metabolic phenotypes) is one that takes into account the complexity of health care and where our model needs to go. Here is my theory of how the medical model should look:

A Multi Factorial Design for the Etiology of Disease

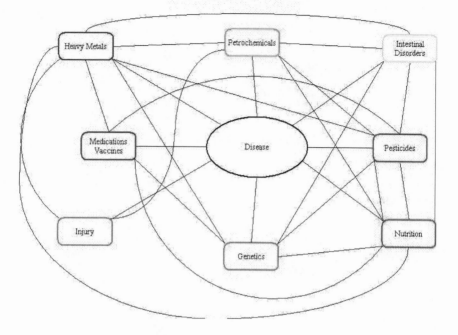

PART III

22. ACHIEVING TRUE VICTORY OVER A TOXIC WORLD

IS THERE REALLY ANY HOPE?

> *"The problems of victory are more agreeable than the problems of defeat, but they are no less difficult."*
>
> Sir Winston Churchill

> *"The moment of victory is much too short to live for that and nothing else."*
>
> Martina Navratilova

> *"Zum Erstaunen ich bin da"*
>
> *– I am here to wonder.*
> Johann Wolfgang von Goethe

My dear friend Robert Crayhon told me that while my lectures were stirring and met with real enthusiasm, the one problem he sees is that many of my talks have a doom and gloom theme to them. You must admit that it is quite difficult to keep a positive outlook when all you seemingly read about is what affects all of the toxins we dump into our world are having on us. The easy way is to let the bad news take over your life and lead you into the dark abyss of depression.

Is it really possible? Can we create an environment that will allow us and our offspring to not only survive but to thrive? Is there really any hope?

My answer is a very timid yes and at the same time a resounding YES.

Over my lifetime, the one accusation lobbed against me has never been one of being negative. If anything has been typical of my attitude it has been an overly exuberant optimism. But, after Tasya's battles, the frustration of watching opinionated, over-educated, and steel trap minded medical "experts" make judgments similar to ones a bartender would make after closing when concocting a new mixed drink, you can imagine my ebullience was somewhat dampened about our world. Still, I cannot give up on people. I will not give up on people. There is a lot of hope out there. What we need to do is make sure we keep the fires kindled under those of us who can spread the word.

The message I want to propose to everyone is that this is not a lost cause. We have not come to a point of no return. Oh, far from it. There is so much we can do to make a difference, as individuals and even as small groups. It does not take a million voices yelling at once saying that we "won't take it anymore." All it takes is each and every one of you to choose to do things that make a difference each day, in your everyday lives. It is not hard, or even inconvenient. To make a difference it does take the one thing that our culture seems to have sadly abandoned: responsibility.

Giving a damn about throwing a granola bar wrapper on the floor is an important first step. The most annoying people to me are those who claim to care so much (enter sarcastic tone of voice) and yet do those thoughtless things that can make such a big difference in achieving an ultimate victory. Eating granola bars and going to Earth Day marches mean little when you throw your crap out the car window for someone else to clean up.

By doing those little things in our lives and teaching our children, we can begin to change the world around us. By making our feelings known, by voting to not buy products that are environmentally unsafe, we can begin to have a greater and greater effect.

If you think it cannot be done, look at the quantity of trans/hydrogenated fats in foods and how quickly they are disappearing from our supermarket shelves (although 7-11s seem to be their last bastion). It did not take people screaming and threatening others, it took the vote of the wallet. Cities like New York are even banning trans fats from restaurants.

Organic foods in the 80s? 90s? Pretty hard to find outside of a health food store. Today organic food is the fastest growing segment of most grocery stores. People are demanding it and getting it. No protests necessary here.

Smoking is another example. In the 70s you were lucky to have a non-smoking section in a restaurant. Now, cities are banning it everywhere including outdoors. Why? Because we demanded it.

Thimerasol in vaccines. It was being used until parents of children with autism demanded that it be removed. The CDC and the FDA swear that it has no correlation with the neurological disease but they removed it anyway. Why? We demanded it.

Why can't we continue and demand that manufacturers use less toxic chemicals? Why can't we demand that our cosmetics no longer contain dangerous chemicals? We are and it is changing.

Is it fast enough? Do we care enough? The answer to both of those questions is sadly no. It isn't fast enough and we don't seem to care enough. The evidence is in how we vote and how many of us vote for officials who are not putting the issue of environmental toxicity at the head of their agendas. Also, how many of us shop as though we cared (cosmetics, nail polish, bleach-free recycled products, etc.)?

I refuse to get into a political debate because neither party in America is doing anything but giving us the lip service they think we deserve. People are not asking loudly enough. We do not need marches and protests we need phone calls and letters. We need blog sites that point out the wrongs of the world. Having worked for a number of politicians many years ago, I knew that when the voters demanded action the politician reacted. It did not take many calls or letters, just enough to get attention.

But what we need more than anything is personal responsibility. To paraphrase the late President John F. Kennedy – 'Ask not what your world can do for you, ask how you can do things to change your world.' Don't yell about it, do it.

Refuse to buy weed killers. Pick the weed out of the ground yourself. Don't complain about thimerasol in your child's vaccines when you don't give a damn about using perfumes high in phthalates because it makes you feel and smell good.

Stop complaining about how polluted your city is when you drive around in a gas guzzling, supersized SUVs. If you drink a case of beer a day, stop whining about your beer belly.

TAKE RESPONSIBILITY. Do it at home first. If I sound somewhat preachy, you're absolutely right. Sometimes you need to shout things out to get heard.

Now say you have done all those things. You have cut your exposures down dramatically and you are making a conscious effort to buy the right products. How do you go about getting rid of what you have in your body already and are being subjected to from others? That is what the rest of this section of the book is about.

23. The Precautionary Principle – The Way Out of Our Toxic Mess?

"Something made greater by ourselves and in turn that makes us greater."

Maya Angelou

"Far and away the best prize that life offers is the chance to work hard at work worth doing."

Theodore Roosevelt

"The world has not to be put in order; the world is order incarnate. It is for us to put ourselves in unison with this order."

Henry Miller

In the 1970s, the West German government was dealing with an issue known as *Waldsterben* or 'forest death'. The famous Black Forest was dying as were other forests that dotted the landscape. Scientists and policy-makers finally understood the calamity that was being caused in part because of air pollution. They needed a way to develop a policy that would help them deal with the immediate issue and with problems yet to come. In 1974 they came up with the *Vorsorgeprinzip* a.k.a. the foresight or precautionary principle.[110]

In medicine and public health, we use this idea all the time. With the possibility of a bird flu pandemic, public health officials are gearing up for the potential which may or may not come about. By using the precautionary principle, they may avert a catastrophic loss of life by preparing for the potential of a crisis and by doing so they may prevent a greater loss of life than if nothing were done at all.

So what is the Precautionary Principle? According to the "Wingspread Statement on the Precautionary Principle" it is:

When an activity raises threats of harm to human health or the environment, precautionary measures should be taken even if some cause and effect relationships are not fully established scientifically.

In this context the proponent of an activity, rather than the public, should bear the burden of proof.

The process of applying the Precautionary Principle must be open, informed and democratic and must include potentially affected parties. It must also involve an examination of the full range of alternatives, including no action.[111]

When the authors of this manifesto talk about openness it is important that the public is made aware of what is going on in their neighborhood. An example is the Toxics Release Inventory, a publicly available database that publishes information on all toxic releases from industry and government. It is accessible from the EPA (Environmental Protection Agency) website at http://epa.gov/tri/. Unfortunately, the current administration is trying to curtail the amount of information going into the database claiming that it is an undo burden on business. What about the undo burden on personal health and well-being? The need to know seriously outweighs the small cost necessary to be good environmental citizens.

According to a great book edited by Nancy J Meyers and Carolyn Raffensperger, *Precautionary Tools for Reshaping*

Environmental Policy, there is a simple, yet complete checklist that can be applied to the decision making process when assessing risks using the Precautionary Principle. There are six basic questions that should be asked:

1. What do we care about?
2. What are we trying to accomplish?
3. What choices do we have?
4. What is the bigger picture?
5. Do we know enough to act? Do we know so little we must act with caution?
6. Who is responsible?

Think about these six items and think about each and how they can make you change the way you act in your everyday life.

The first one should make you evaluate what your values are in life. What do you really care about? Is it your livelihood at the risk of your health? Is it the environment that your children and grandchildren will be left with? By answering this question we will be better suited to understand what we want to do.

What we want to do is known as a goal, and goals as Nancy Meyers says "...are powerful instruments."[112] Goals are like beacons that shine in the distance that draw us to them and as we move towards them we realize that there are many paths, some easy, some difficult, each with different repercussions. This brings us to the next item, and that is answering what choices we have.

Each of us has to choose what risks and concessions we are willing to take in order to reach our goal. This goes back to what your values are. It also means that you have to make decisions as to what impact your choice will have on others. Sometimes the decision is easy, like choosing to bring a reusable bag to the supermarket instead of being asked "plastic or paper." Others decisions are more difficult, like demanding the closing of a manufacturing plant that is polluting the environment but supplies jobs to your community.

While looking at all the options, you may need to look outside the box and look for paths that may not be apparent or you may need to blaze a new one. The decision is yours. But still, you need to look at the bigger picture when making a choice of where to go.

There are times when the decision to go in one direction towards the goal you set forth actually takes you on a course that contains unwanted repercussions. There are numerous cases where intervening in our environment without looking at the bigger picture caused more harm than good. Sometimes, not doing anything or acting with extreme caution will bring us closer to our goal than hastily reacting.

This issue deals with question number five which should cause us to look at our environment, look at the path we chose and observe our steps carefully so we can catch ourselves before we do something harmful. We can always go back easier if we have not gone that far forward. One step backwards is easier than ten.

When looking at our path, we need to be cognizant of bias in determining harm or benefit. In a case in Mexico, concerned citizens complained that scientists who cautioned about a problem of gene transfer to native plants from genetically modified plants were somehow biased in their research. When looking deeper into whom these "concerned" people were they turned out to be a public relations firm hired by the producer of the genetically modified plants, Monsanto.[113] This is why freedom of information is our best guardian and should be protected at all costs.

And finally, we need to assess who is truly responsible for what is going on and who is responsible for getting us to our final destination, our goal. We need to find out who is responsible for the problems, who is responsible for fixing the problem (government, private sector or private citizens) and how are we going to get to the goal that is economically, socially and logically sound. Once we do that, the achievement of our goals are set, and we can turn this downward spiral around. Our environment and our health can be saved and improved.

24. The Top 10 Things You Can Do in the Face of a Toxic World

"An ounce of action is worth a ton of theory."

Friedrich Engels

"The shortest answer is doing."

English proverb

"A human action becomes genuinely important when it springs from the soil of a clear-sighted awareness of the temporality and the ephemerality of everything human. It is only this awareness that can breathe any greatness into an action."

Vaclav Havel

While lecturing at Medicine Week in Baden Baden, Germany in October 2005, a reporter from Chile asked me to list the top ten things that one should do to prevent the effects of toxicity in today's environment. I was able to list eight pretty quickly which satisfied her curiosity but it made me think. What would the top ten things be?

Finally I came up with ten items that everyone should strive to do in order to give themselves a chance to achieve victory over a toxic world.

Here they are:

10 – Don't Let Your Plastic Bottle Get Hot

9 – Drink Enough Fluids

8 – Sweat

7 – Laboratory Testing

6 – Get Rid of Your Mercury Fillings

5 – Detox Heavy Metals

4 – Increase Glutathione Production and Make Glycine Part of Your Life

3 – Never Microwave Food and Plastics Together

2 – Get Educated and Get Involved

1 – Lower Your Use and Practice Avoidance

#10 – Don't Let Your Plastic Bottle Get Hot

Leaving your plastic water bottle in your car in the summer, then drinking from it is a superb way of ingesting toxins, especially phthalates. Keeping them in direct sunlight is another marvelous way to increase toxin intake.

I have been asked about whether freezing a plastic bottle does the same as heating it. My answer is that there is no evidence that freezing releases toxins. From what I have seen, this is actually an internet hoax that claims that researchers from Johns Hopkins University found that plastic bottles release dioxin when frozen. This never happened, yet, as is typical with the internet, the myth spreads unchecked.

#9 – Drink Enough Fluids

Since most people are so fluid deficient, they obviously cannot excrete most toxins in either their sweat or urine. Now, when I talk fluids, I do not just mean water. I also do not mean increasing your alcohol or coffee intake as well; those are classified as diuretics and will deplete your fluid level. What I do mean is that you need to get a wide variety of fluids into yourself all day long.

The problem I see with water is that while it is a great dissolver of toxins, you have to remember that it is the universal solvent and it will cause nutrients to be washed away as well. Excessive water can lead to nutrient depletion so whenever possible, drink water with some mineralization.

Mix your fluids intake up and make sure that you take adequate electrolytes (not Gatorade® or PowerAde® please). Make sure you use high quality electrolytes that do not contain unnecessary sugars, such as Crayhon Research's Peltier, which I formulated because what is out on the market is not what you should be putting in your body if you want to improve fluid levels.

Here is a quick test of whether you have an adequate fluid level. Sit down on a chair with your hand on your lap face down. Look at the back of your hands, they should have puffy veins sticking out (if not, you are severely dehydrated). Slowly bring your hand up always looking at the veins. Note when they disappear. If it is below eye level, you are fluid deficient. If they disappear at chest level, you are about a quart low.

Another way to determine if you are fluid deficient is if you get dizzy when you stand up quickly from a seated position. It usually means (although not always) that you do not have enough fluids to reach your brain. Some people at this point swear they drink enough but when you start to review their actual intake over a long period of time, they usually do not drink enough on a day to day basis.

#8 – Sweat

Sweating is one of the best ways to release toxins and improve circulation. There are many ways to induce sweating including exercise and saunas. There is a debate going around over the usefulness of far infrared saunas (FIR) and whether they really are safe and effective. I have heard both sides of the argument and so far the best FIR I can recommend is by Heavenly Heat Contact: Bob Morgan, Owner, Heavenly Heat Saunas, P.O. Box 2892, Crested Butte, CO 81224, Ph: 1-800-697-2862,

Still, the overwhelming information about the benefits of sauna comes from the use of traditional saunas so the use of FIRs in detoxification is somewhat theoretical but it does have the potential for definite benefits.

One comment I read that I think is apropos to include here is one made by Dr. Andy Cutler about sweating at night being a sign of mercury intoxication. Night sweats are a common problem with toxic individuals and should be looked into further through the use of the next tip that will help you deal with a toxic world – Laboratory Testing.

#7 – Laboratory Testing

Interpreting laboratory tests is my primary business so it may come as a surprise that it shows up at only #7 in the list of things to do to help deal with a toxic world. The reason is simple, while I feel that assessing what types of environmental insults are making you unhealthy, doing the other nine things is just as important.

Now don't get me wrong, getting tested is essential. Finding out what you are dealing with is the way to determine the appropriate treatments. Without testing, you are playing in the dark and can cause damage to your health.

An example would be the different strategies necessary to detoxify benzene versus styrene. With benzene if you detoxify improperly before working on your gut flora (probiotic therapy) you can create phenolic compounds which can cause benzene to become carcinogenic while with styrene, this issue is not that critical.

You also need to know the health of your gut. Is it filed with pathogenic bacteria? If so, then your ability to completely detoxify will be severely impaired. The use of probiotics as a regular daily regimen should be part of your everyday routine, but if the laboratory testing shows high levels of pathogenic bacteria then appropriate action is necessary. In some cases, antibiotic therapy may be called for. Of course, only a qualified physician can suggest this.

Here is a tip from the files of my brain; when using antibiotics it may be beneficial to use ammonium chloride adjunctively to prevent secondary infections. How do I come about this information? Well, good old John Kitkoski showed me a book that was printed around 1947 or so. It had a passage where they recommended the use of this inexpensive compound to prevent secondary yeast infections which may occur in some people due to the use of antibiotics. He then showed me the following year's version of the book where all that was changed was that one passage. The change was that instead of using ammonium chloride, it recommended using Nystatin (an anti-fungal) if a secondary infection occurs. Don't prevent it when you can cure it after you get it. Makes sense eh? Didn't think so.

To get more information about this topic, go to the chapter on laboratory testing for chronic conditions.

#6 – GET RID OF YOUR MERCURY FILLINGS

The American Dental Association may want you to believe that the amalgam fillings you have in your mouth are safe and that there is no evidence that they cause any health issues but I am here to tell you that it is absolutely in your best interest to get them out. Mercury is one of the most toxic substances known to man and any amount whether so-called inert or not is just not worth having in your body. This is doubly true if you are a genetic non-excretor of mercury (see my discussion about Apolipoprotein E).

Having said that, you have to make sure that the dentist you use is very well trained in how to do this safely. The last thing you need is to remove amalgam fillings from your mouth and in the process inhale the fumes or ingest tiny bits and pieces of mercury.

More information about this subject can be gathered from Dr. Andrew Cutler's book, *Amalgam Illness* (available from www. noamalgam.com). It is not an easy read, and it is not written to entertain, but it does have important information about mercury amalgams that everyone should know about. Which leads us to our next tip.......

#5 – Detoxify Heavy Metals

The detoxification of heavy metals is a critical next step in order to achieve optimal health. Having said that, detoxifying the wrong way is dangerous, as I have seen enough people get seriously messed up because of it. I have also seen more products that tout their ability to detoxify metals that just are not real.

This subject is one that could easily make me a battalion of enemies by naming those products that are more efficacious at removing money from your wallet than metals from your body. There are a lot of hucksters that are making some big money at the expense of the public. Instead of exposing them I will comment on the methodology that I feel works best. Understand that my omission of a particular detox method or product does not mean that it is quackery, just that I feel the following is superior.

The use of low dose oral, **not** intravenous (IV), DMSA (dimercaptosuccinic acid) on an every four hour dosage with a three day on, four day off protocol with alpha lipoic acid, Peltier electrolytes (see resources at the end of the book), vitamin C (as well as other antioxidants) and trace minerals will give you the most bang for the buck and is the safest way to remove mercury. If you are looking to remove lead, EDTA (ethylenediaminetetraacetic acid) tops the charts. For the other metals, I suggest you pick up Dr. Cutler's book as this becomes a very involved topic.

#4 – Increase Glutathione Production
and Make Glycine Part of Your Life

Fellow colleague Dr. Dietrich Klinghardt once told me that because of information from my lectures he had begun adding 1000 milligrams of glycine to every one of his patient's daily regimes. In light of the enormous amount of solvents that we are subjected to every day, I have to concur with his recommendation as glycine is used by the body to conjugate (bind) intermediary detoxification compounds that if left alone are oftentimes more toxic than the original substance.

Glycine is, thankfully, one of the least expensive nutritional supplements around. It is neuroinhibitory (calming) and has some other remarkable benefits like being able to be converted to serine which helps build the neurotransmitter acetyl choline, critical in the functioning of short term memory.

Another nice benefit of this powerhouse nutrient is in the treatment of gout. Instead of sending their patient to the pharmacy to fill in a prescription for allopurinol, the physician should start them off with a gram of glycine a day. I have given this tip to a few physician friends and one was thrilled as it made her husband who was suffering from the tell tale achy foot better in just a couple of days.

As for glutathione, there are a number of controversies surrounding the best way to boost it in the body. I wish I had the definitive answer for you, but as always, I will give you my opinion on the subject. If you need a quick boost, stay away from the IV. Try a combination of vitamin C 500 milligrams twice a day, selenium 200 mcg and an amino acid complex like My Aminoplex from Crayhon Research (775-823-5333 professionals only). Dr. David Quig of Doctor's Data laboratories swears by whey protein as a great way to boost glutathione production. Others would disagree with that recommendation as they say that some people are sensitive to the high sulfur in the product.

Some suggest reduced glutathione as a way to get by the problem of absorption as straight glutathione is too large of a molecule to get absorbed in the gut.

#3 – Never Microwave Food and Plastics Together

There are those out there who would say that you should never microwave anything, and I can't say that I totally disagree with them. Microwaving foods is just another way to bypass the time tested cooking methods which humankind has used for a millennium and adds to our culture of being the "land of instant pudding". Our rush to do everything stops us from enjoying food and having a sit down dinner with our family to recount our daily activities, but I digress.

Think of microwaving food wrapped in plastic as a way of infusing the chemicals used to make the plastic into our food. I don't know about you but I sure don't think that sounds very appealing nor should it. Styrene and phthalates add very little nutritionally to our foods and certainly do not make it taste any better.

This hint should include any heating of plastics from leaving your plastic water bottle in the car on a hot day (see tip #10) to drinking hot coffee or tea from a Styrofoam cup. Heat plus plastics equals a bad idea. If you need to use the microwave, do so with the food on a glass or ceramic (not made with heavy metal containing glazes) plate or cup. Better yet, allow your microwave to gather dust and not use it at all.

#2 – Get Educated and Get Involved

Reading this book is a step towards education and going through the reference section will guide you towards other educational websites, books, and journals that will help you become better educated on the field of environmental toxicity. By being better educated you can make wiser decisions regarding day-to-day activities and lifestyle choices that will keep you, your family and your friends healthier and happier.

As for involvement, there are varying degrees that have to coincide with what you feel comfortable with. Not everyone wants to set up a large-scale protest against environmental polluters or begin a letter writing campaign. Others would feel deprived if all they did was to make changes in their purchasing habits and daily activities. Neither one is better than the other. Everything you do to change the environment around you, whether you decide to stop purchasing products that are toxic, to writing your elected officials, to going out and protesting the use of thimerasol in vaccines, are all important steps in making a global change in how we treat our world.

A case in point is the change in the use of trans-fats in potato chips and other snack foods. Just recently, many of the major food companies like Frito Lays and General Foods started marketing trans-fat free products. The lettering on their packaging heralding the improvements was bold and big and trumpeted the fact that they were concerned about the health of their product.

A few of you may be a wee bit skeptical with the idea that this was done out of good intentions and that the big food manufacturers were turning a new leaf and had our health in mind when they made the switch to non-hydrogenated fats. I will join you in that hefty bit of skepticism and say that the reason for the changes was the protest we made with our wallets/pocketbooks. Sales were sagging and publicity was starting to get negative so they were forced to make the change. No one started a Million Mom March to force this change. There were no burning bags of corn chips lining the streets; it was our dollars that did the talking.

If we stop buying microwavable plastic lunches, if we stop paying money for cans lined with bisphenol A, and if we decide that we don't want coffee in Styrofoam cups, then we will slowly make a difference in this world. Each little step begets another.

#1 – LOWER YOUR USE AND AVOID, AVOID, AVOID

Basically this tip is an accumulation of all of the previous tips plus more. It is the most important one of all, though. If you do everything else, educate, detox, remove your amalgams, drink lots of fluids, stop using your microwave, and all of the other tips and suggestions throughout the book and you do not work at avoiding all the other toxic insults, then you run the risk of unwinding all of the other things you have done to improve your health.

Work hard at looking around your home and office and get rid of as many items as you can that will increase your toxic exposure. Follow some of the ideas I will present in the coming chapters, most of which are relatively easy to follow.

25. TIME: The Forgotten Nutrient

"We must use time as a tool, not as a couch."

John F. Kennedy

"For tribal man, space was the uncontrollable mystery. For technological man it is time that occupies the same role."

Marshall McLuhan

"Time and I against any two."

Spanish proverb

America is the land of instant pudding. We want everything now, not tomorrow, not next week or next year, but right this very minute. There is an expectation that we don't need to wait for anything anymore due to our accelerated technological advances. We are such an impatient country that we fail to appreciate important things in life until they are long gone, especially when it comes to our health.

A common complaint I hear from many health care practitioners is that while drug therapies have an immediate impact, nutritional ones take too long and this causes them to lose patients who do not want to wait for results. I have a real problem with this because all it takes is simply educating the patient and making them understand the concept of time. This chapter is an attempt to show you how to use time and understand its value in the process of achieving optimal health.

One thing I want to be clear about is that there are many instances where time is truly of the essence, where immediate intervention is critical and patience is unwarranted. One such case involves a child's health, especially with autism.

The autistic child is one, who in my opinion, has been environmentally abused. The use of thimerasol and the subsequent cover-up is an exhibit of the worst in humankind. The denial of mercury amalgams causing health problems is equally disconcerting. The proper and complete chelation of mercury from adults' and children's brains is not one where time can wait. Each passing day that a nanogram of mercury is allowed to continue to destroy neurons in the brain is one day too many.

According to numerous accounts I've seen on Yahoo newsgroups such as ABMD (Autism Biomedical) and Autism-Mercury, autistic children have made incredible improvements using proper chelation therapies. Dr. Andrew Cutler also reports on the numerous benefits of chelating mercury in his book *Amalgam Illness*. He makes a comment which I think is quite apropos when talking about detoxifying children – "Don't lose your golden opportunity by waiting!" Dr. Cutler is pretty adamant that the time to chelate is before adolescence and not to wait because of fear and confusion.

But it is his comment in the beginning of the book that I want to focus on:

> *"It takes a while to get better. Even if you do everything perfectly. Be realistic. Prepare yourself, your plans, your job and your finances for a rough year or two. Tell your friends and family it is going to be a rough time and you will need their help. Count on the ones who indicate they understand and act like they want to help. Don't fool yourself into depending on people because they are "supposed" to help. Depend on the ones who are WILLING to help, regardless of who is supposed to."[114]*

His comment is quite profound in today's world. Our family structures have changed so much over the years that the strong bonds that kept us together and helped support us through tough times have eroded. One of the great tragedies I have witnessed is the disintegration of marriages in families with neurologically challenged children, especially the families of autistic children. The patience to be **willing** to be supportive disappears in the face of adversity. The inability to understand the concept of time as it relates to health is so prevalent. Sadly, it is the male member of the couple who most often abandons the family (although I have heard cases of mothers taking the healthy kids and leaving the autistic one with the husband).

But it is not just the lack of patience in helping others that is a problem in today's modern society, it is the lack of patience to help oneself and take the time to rebuild and restructure one's chemistry that is problematic. In my opinion, it is one of the reasons for the explosive growth of the pharmaceutical industry. It isn't just the flashy marketing or the constant rep whose visits to the doctor's office that are solely to blame. It is our impatience and demand for immediate reactions and solutions that are also at fault. We do not want a solution to the problem, we want to cover it up and make it go away.

I think it is critical for the health care practitioner to talk about time and how it needs to be thought of as a nutrient. While chemical reactions occur in nanoseconds billions of times a day in our bodies, Rome wasn't built in a day nor was your body. Think of how long it took for you to get the way that you are. Short of an accident or a infection, most illnesses are due to long-term behavior or exposures. When talking toxicity, usually it is not the one time contact that causes you problems but many exposures to numerous toxic agents.

It is the lack of understanding this concept that allows many of the polluters and industry apologists to get away with things. If the reaction does not occur right away, it does not happen in their eyes. The idea of a chain of events happening because of numerous exposures to stress, toxins, and infections that directs a person's chemistry towards ill health is how we should be looking at disease creation. It is the use of biochemically individualized nutritional and behavioral protocols over an extended period of time that will reverse the negative chain of events and hopefully redirect the biochemistry to a positive direction that will allow the individual to achieve their goal of not only the lack of disease but the attainment of optimal health.

26. Common Sense (and not so apparent) Tips to Improve Our Environment

"Common sense is the measure of the possible; it is composed of experience and prevision; it is calculation applied to life."

Henri Fredric Amiel

"All truth, in the long run, is only common sense clarified."

Thomas Henry Huxley

"Common sense always speaks too late. Common sense is the guy who tells you you ought to have had your breaks relined last week before you smashed a front end this week. Common sense is the Monday morning quarterback who could have won the ball game if he had been on the team.

> *But he never is. He's high up in the stands with a flask on his hip. Common sense is the little man in a grey suit who never makes a mistake in addition. But it's always somebody else's money he's adding up."*

> *Raymond Chandler*

Common sense is something always in short supply but seemingly easy to come by. When it comes to making differences in our environment and improving our world what seems to be logical isn't always so. Take for instance the idea of replacing incandescent light bulbs with fluorescent bulbs.

A fluorescent bulb contains trace amounts of mercury while incandescents do not but it would be prudent to make the change in part to *reduce* mercury emissions. How is this possible? It doesn't make common sense. Or does it?

According to Dr. Bill Chameides, chief scientist at the Environmental Defense Fund (www.environmentaldefense.org) it's an easy answer. Because a fluorescent bulb uses so much less energy, if every household in America were to switch three bulbs to the more efficient light source it would be the equivalent of removing 3.5 million cars from the road. Also, by reducing energy use it would lower the emissions of mercury from coal burning plants by enough to counter the minute amount of mercury in each bulb. If you can, swap out all of your incandescent bulbs to make up for all of the people who won't heed this advice.

One other comment is important here and that is to make sure you do not dump used fluorescent bulbs into the regular garbage; it should be handled in the hazardous waste disposal system which most larger communities have.

So common sense tip #1 is

> *Replace at least three incandescent light bulbs with fluorescent light bulbs.*

Recycling is a hot issue on both sides with proponents touting the resource issue and the opponents claiming that it is too expensive. In actuality, the reason recycling is not as cost effective as it should be is because of the small number of people who recycle. In Pittsburgh, Pennsylvania where only seven percent of the people recycle the cost per ton was $470 whereas in communities where the recycling rate was closer to twenty percent their cost per ton was a more reasonable $93.[115] But this should not even be the issue. Our environment should be and time and time again research has shown that recycling reduces energy use and lowers many kinds of air and water pollution. Just with aluminum alone we know that it takes twenty five percent less energy to produce cans from recycled materials than virgin ore.[116]

COMMON SENSE TIP #2

Recycle. Don't complain, just do it.

The single most wasteful place when it comes to the environment is your home. As I mentioned in the first tip, changing a few light bulbs can be helpful but what about the rest of the house? Refrigerators are the #1 energy sucking device so wouldn't it make sense that when the time comes to buy a new one, you find the most energy efficient one? That and tell the kids to not stand in front of the fridge with the door wide open while they swig a drink of juice.

Buy a front-load washer. Not only do they use less water per load than a top load washer (14 versus 40 gallons), the newer models spin dry clothes faster meaning the dryer time is reduced considerably saving more energy.

Let's think about the water savings for a moment. Say that the cost of water per gallon is .004 cents. If you think about it that's 10.4 cents of savings per load. If we do 4 loads a week (if you have a really neat family) that comes out to a savings of $21.62 a year. Now that may not seem like much but when you realize you saved 5,408 gallons of water, you can see how important that is. Imagine if 100,000 people bought a front-load versus a top load last year. We would have saved 5.4 billion gallons of water!!!

Look around your home and see where you can cut back on energy use. Turn off those night lights, insulate around windows, lower the thermostat temperature to 68°F during the winter and raise it during the summer to 78° F, and when buying appliances make the energy use the most important factor in your purchase decision. Not only is this good for the environment but its good for the national economy (lowers our dependence of foreign fuel). It can save you and your family thousands of dollars a year.

COMMON SENSE TIP #3

Do an energy survey of your house and make reducing your daily use a family priority.

Feeding people is another enormous drain on resources. As many people know, I am neither a light eater nor do I espouse radical eating habits but there are two simple things you can do that is both healthy and good for the environment and that is to eat less red meat and whenever possible, buy organically grown foods. This may seem obvious but the impact is greater than you might think.

Here are a few facts about meat consumption from the excellent book "*The Consumer's Guide to Effective Environmental Choices*" by Michael Brower and Warren Leon, both members of the Union of Concerned Scientists:[117]

- 18% of water consumption in the U.S. is to grow feed for livestock.
- 16% of water quality problems are directly attributable to animal waste.
- 2 billion pounds of wet manure is generated annually which is ten times the amount us humans put out.
- 40% of the U.S. land mass or 800 million acres are used for livestock grazing.

As you can see, meat production is a huge drain on resources. Cattle account for forty five percent of the waste production, chickens representing thirty four percent, and pigs twelve percent. So cutting down on red meat consumption does have a positive effect.

Lest you vegetarians out there think your consumption does not affect the environment, think again. The water use surrounding the growing of fruits, vegetables and grains is a staggering thirty percent. Add to that the use of fertilizers, pesticides, and soil erosion and you can see how this presents a problem. But there is a solution and that is to buy only certified organic fruits, vegetables and grain products whenever possible. There is quite a bit of evidence that organic farming techniques are less demanding of resources and more obviously they use far less toxic chemicals like pesticides than conventional farming does. Yes, there is a premium cost involved in buying organic but if we make this choice and more people demand it, the price will eventually come down.

COMMON SENSE TIP #4

Eat less red meat and buy certified organic foods whenever possible.

Weight watching is on everyone's mind today but the weight I'm about to talk about has nothing to do with dieting, it has to do with how you look at your day to day actions to protect the environment. One of my mantras is to not sweat the small stuff and concentrate on big issues. If we spend a lot of our energy worrying about whether to use plastic bags or paper at the grocery store (there is very little difference actually) but we drive a gas guzzling SUV all the time there is something mightily wrong here. The big, heavy car will have a lot more impact than a year's worth of little plastic bags. Focus on the big issues like buying a more efficient car, refrigerator, or even desk for your office, than the little issues. Buying a lighter desk is environmentally more efficient than buying a heavier one.

I may get a bit of guff about this but let me clarify things. I get a bit irked at places that put two or three items into a plastic bag instead of a more reasonable amount but I don't spend a lot of time on it. What I spent this year doing was investigating the purchase of a hybrid vehicle which beyond the great gas mileage, it puts out 90% fewer emissions than does a regular gas powered vehicle and considerably less than a big SUV or truck. My wife and I spent more time looking at a front-loading washer than worrying about using plastic or glass bottles although it was important to look at all of the issues. There is a real finite amount of time that anyone can give to making environmentally safe choices and we need to spend that time efficiently. If we make a too much noise about insignificant issues that have little impact we may miss the big items that make way more of a difference.

COMMON SENSE TIP #5

When making decisions about environmental impact, be a weight watcher. The heavier the item, the more impact it has and the more time you should spend on making a decision about it.

Guilt, ah, an American way of being. We feel so much guilt over so many things we sometimes get mired in the morass of it all. As I mentioned previously, do not sweat the little stuff. Let's add a little corollary; do not feel guilty about the little stuff either.

What do I mean about not feeling guilty? I mean don't feel bad that you chose disposable diapers versus cloth because there is little evidence that one is better or worse than the other. The argument for cloth diapers is that they don't clog landfills and don't produce as many toxic chemicals in their production and destruction. Disposable diaper users point to the lowered use of water in cleaning which in turn uses less energy which is better for the environment. So who is right? Neither and both but if you read down a little further, you will see there really is a difference but it isn't for an obvious reason. Environmentally speaking, it's a draw so don't spend much time on the discussion and concentrate on bigger environmental issues.

Here are a few others to not feel guilty about:

- Paper or Plastic bags – It's really a draw between these two. If you really are concerned, get a cloth bag and reuse that. Otherwise, move on.
- Cotton or synthetic clothing – Both use resources and both have issues but the difference isn't that great. Make your choice based on fashion and not on environmental impact.
- Paper packing material or synthetic "peanuts" – Guess what? Another non-issue. Paper weighs more which means it uses more resources which causes toxic releases (remember to be a weight watcher), peanuts are more toxic themselves but weigh less. No real difference here either.

Here is one to feel guilty about:

- Disposable diapers versus Reusable cloth diapers – Sorry to say, this is a slam dunk on the side of cloth diapers. First off, the average cloth diaper is equivalent to 170 disposable ones. Secondly, when the disposable diaper hits the landfill, the bacteria, viruses, and other pathogens that may linger in the fecal matter or urine could make their way to groundwater supplies. With cloth, the waste would go through water treatment plants which are built to handle the pathogens.[118]

Bottom line is to avoid getting your shorts in a bunch about things that aren't going to make a real impact.

Common sense tip #6

Don't feel overly guilty about small issues regarding the environment, concentrate on important issues.

One comment I hear a lot is how little each of us can really do in the greater scheme of things. It is a comment that makes me cringe somewhat. If we really look at many of the incredible world changing events we see that it oftentimes begins with just a handful of people making some noise. The movement away from trans fats in foods didn't start with a million man march. It started with some people who demanded better.

When I was a boy of 12 way back in 1970, I started a recycling program on West 89th Street in Manhattan, New York. It blossomed from there and now millions of people set out their recycling bins. Now I'm not claiming to have started the movement, but as a little kid I helped push things along. Each of us can do the same.

Choose not to use pesticides and other chemicals around your home, choose to consume less and make choices that are eco-friendly. If each one of us decides to make better choices and tell our friends and families about it without being smug, you would be amazed at the kind of effect you will have and how the world will change.

COMMON SENSE TIP #7

You can make a big difference in this world. No change is too insignificant. Start today and the world will change.

Here is a list of down and dirty, quick and easy things to improve your footprint on our environment.

- Bag the use of air fresheners. If you absolutely must use one, try Pure Citrus Orange Air Freshener by Pure Citrus, Inc. out of Kennesaw, GA.
- Don't store chemicals under the sink where hot water pipes can impart enough heat to volatilize the compounds into the air you breathe.
- I'll say it one more time; don't heat or microwave anything stored in or covered with plastic.
- Don't use chlorine bleach. Suffer through slightly less white socks and underwear. Use non-chlorine bleach instead.
- Buy frozen or fresh food instead of canned. This will lower your exposure to that nasty toxin bisphenol A.
- If you can, buy paper that is either unbleached or doesn't use chlorine in processing.
- If you have to have your clothes dry cleaned, let them air dry for two days before wearing them. Better yet, don't dry clean your clothes and use Dryel® instead. It isn't perfect but it is less toxic than dry cleaning.
- Try buying eco-safe laundry detergents from your local health food store. They may be more expensive but they do make a big difference. They use less phosphates and do less damage to the environment.
- Choose products with pumps rather than aerosol sprays. Aerosol sprays have been implicated in depletion of the ozone layer.
- Look for products that say biodegradable and/or recyclable whenever possible.

If each person who reads this book follows the six main tips and ten quickies from this chapter, the world will be a better place in which to live in and by leading by example, you will have many followers. The world can change one household at a time. It has to start somewhere.

27. Opinions: Yes I Have a Few.....

"Opinions are to the vast apparatus of social existence what oil is to machines: one does not go up to a turbine and pour machine oil over it; one applies a little to hidden spindles and joints that one has to know."

Walter Benjamin

"Opinions are made to be changed – or how is truth to be got at?"

Lord Byron

"New opinions are always suspected, and usually opposed, without any other reason but because they are not already common."

John Locke

One of the problems I will never have is lacking an opinion. After spending the past 20+ years researching health issues, I feel that I have earned a right to have an opinion about a number of issues. What

I don't have is "the" answer to anything. Nor, in my opinion, does anyone else. Let me explain.

Ptolemy, in his work the *Almagest*, wrote that the earth was at the center of the universe and everything circled it in concentric globes. This theory ruled as *the truth* until a man named Copernicus came around and developed a *new truth* that had the sun at the center with the earth circling it. This became the new truth in until Johannes Kepler took Tycho Brahe's information and developed a new theory which changed the way we looked at our world yet again. That is until Sir Isaac Newton stood on "the shoulder of Giants" and revolutionized things once more. Then came a small, wild haired man named Albert Einstein who turned the world upside down.

Each one of these brilliant men had an answer but not "the answer". They all had an opinion about what was right, and how things worked. Time and new findings change what we know regularly. Anyone who claims to have found "the only answer" should be avoided at all costs.

We learn, we change, we discover. This is how breakthroughs are made. When we begin to practice in platitudes and absolutes we start the process of walling in our knowledge and we start to build barriers to expand our knowledge that ultimately leads to the world passing us by.

I say all of this because when I have an opinion, it may rub people the wrong way and make them believe that my feet are stuck in cement on the issue. Oh far from it. My fundamental belief is that I only have a small piece of an answer and that I have so much to learn. On the flip side, I have gathered an enormous amount of information and have developed a number of hypotheses that have proven beneficial to many.

The next few chapters relate to a number of issues I think are important to discuss. My goal is not to be boring but also not to be outlandish.

AUTISM AND THE VACCINE ISSUE

Vaccines, in my opinion, do not cause autism. The preservative thimerasol, also, does not cause autism. Before you get ready to lynch me, read on. Both were important triggers that have caused many children to develop autism. This is clear, based on the research and my talks with many parents, researchers, and physicians who have seen many children go from being normal, healthy, and highly interactive to becoming varying degrees of autistic shortly after being vaccinated. To get more information about this I highly recommend reading the book *Evidence of Harm* by David Kirby (that is if you can control your temper – it is very provocative).

Whether it was a genetic quirk (I don't believe that genes can be bad or abnormal – see my opinions about genetics later in this chapter), an unfortunate timing issue, or whatever, vaccines are not the only issue that makes a child autistic. Solvents, other heavy metals (not just mercury), exposure to other toxins during fetal development, abuse, some unknown outside force, or any combination of these may be at the root of the explosion of autism in the world today.

What is important is to look into all of these possibilities because what works for one child may not work for another and in the world of autism, time is truly of the essence. Heavy metal chelation, especially for mercury, may be very important for a high proportion (maybe as high as 76%) of autistic kids.[119] But as a stand alone therapy, it may miss great opportunities. According to Dr. Bernard Rimland's Defeat Autism Now website www.autismwebsite.com/ari/index.htm the simple addition of the supplements magnesium and vitamin B6 had a positive effect on over 47% of children with autism with only 4% showing a negative effect. This data is based upon 5780 reported cases.

Bottom Line: Vaccines are often times the trigger that pulls the loaded gun that is pointed at children with autism, but they are not solely to blame for the explosion in the incidence of autism

I Can Cure Autism

Why write so many opinions on the subject of autism? Because I am struck by the seemingly predatory actions of certain "autism experts" and the way they separate desperate parents from their bank accounts in the guise of helping children. While many of the people out there in the field genuinely care and believe they are doing things in the best interest of the autistic community, I find many of their actions go beyond any sense of moralism or honesty.

When I go to conferences on autism, whether it is AutismOne in the Chicago area, or DAN (Defeat Autism Now), which has numerous conferences coast-to-coast, I am always struck by the flavor-of-the-month speakers, who get up there and espouse that they have "the answer" to autism and that if you pay them only $800 an hour, they will stick a patch of their proprietary blend of carefully researched stuff and your child will be talking like Oprah Winfrey in a few weeks. Read my chapter called the Three Blind Monkey Theory and you will see how some of these people make their money and how they continue to stay in practice for way too many years.

Some of them have truly helped a number of children, and I applaud that and am very happy for the parents of the children (and certainly for the kids themselves). What I have a deep problem with is how they make platitudinal statements that suggest that they, and only they, have the answer that all parents should be banging down their doors to get. Unfortunately, nothing works that way.

There is one doctor who claims that he has cured 30 of 31 children of autism. Or was it 15 of 17? Maybe it was 20 of 22, or 17 of 19. Can't be sure because it seems to change every time I see him or hear his lectures. But soon, the study will be released and the real number will come out (yawn, it's been years of promises of the publication of the study but nothin' yet). Some of you know of whom I speak, some of you don't. I won't mention his name because he is not alone. There are many others out there as guilty, if not more so, of not being completely forthright and making over the top claims.

One famous doctor and I were standing in a hallway discussing each other's talk at a health care conference when he mentioned that his product line was essential in curing autism. I immediately mentioned that the FDA might have a problem with making a claim like that without substantial research data to back him up. His comment back to me was at first puzzling then astonishing. He said "We don't accept anything less than 100% cure of autism."

This comment can be taken a number of ways, but the one that eventually settled in was that we only accept the responses from parents whose children have been "cured" (no definition was given as to what "cured" meant). The reason I say this is when I went to the doctor's own website, and perused his forum, I found that a number of parents were complaining that their kids were not showing much of an improvement on the regimen. The answer they were given was almost always the same, 'can't be our products, it must be something wrong you're doing.'

That last phrase of always blaming the user and not the product is a common one used by people who make outrageous cure rate claims. In my experience over the years, many people who claim to follow a particular recommendation are indeed not doing so, but there are many instances where people are doing everything they have been asked to do and still fail to get the desired response. This happens because we are such unique individuals. Our genes, our environment, our lifestyles all make for a very fluid state of biochemistry not easily and perfectly treatable.

Bottom line: Use the old adage, "If it sounds too good to be true, it is."

GENETICALLY MODIFIED FOOD (GMF) –

DISASTER OR LIFE-SAVING BREAKTHROUGH?

It is debatable as to whether, by genetically modifying food – in which we can breed pest-resistance, increased per-acre yields, and countless other "benefits" into our food supply will help solve world hunger. While the theory seems great, the harsh reality is that geneticists that work for companies like ADM (Archer Daniels Midland) who promote GMF are not taking into account one very important scientific fact: gene-transfers.

According to Heritage (2004)[120] and Netherwood, et al (2004)[121], people who ingest genetically modified foods have caused genes to transfer from the food into the beneficial bacteria in their gut which altered their character. Since many of these friendly bacteria are crucial in digesting our food and creating nutrients from them, what affect will this have on our health and the health of our children?

My friends, we are tinkering with the essence of life and we don't have a clue what we are doing. If we do, then those involved in genetically modifying our foods are up to something nefarious. I hope it is just blind stupidity and greed that guides their hands.

TESTING THE SAFETY OF PESTICIDES ON HUMANS

This is a subject that has recently come under debate and while I find it morally reprehensible, scientifically it makes as much sense as sending a man to the moon in a spaceship built of cheddar cheese. The fact that anyone in the scientific community would somehow think the idea has merit shows the corrupting power of money. To further even remotely suggest that it should be tried not only on males and females but on children and pregnant women should make one compare it to the mind set of the infamous Nazi war criminal Joseph Mengele. This is my main concern but there is equally strong scientific reasoning behind the arguments why not to do human testing.

The rational behind testing humans is that the industry believes it is going to allow for more reasonable uses of pesticides in order to allow farmers to increase production of food and to prevent starvation caused by those nasty critters out there. They further claim that previous methods of safety testing are not allowing us to use the newer generation of chemicals. Scientists (I use this term out of respect for their education, not their ideas) who represent the industry have continually told Congress and the White House that they need to do testing on humans which will show how safe the pesticides are. And guess what? They're right, it will. But it is really a big lie and a way to deceive the public.

Here are my arguments against the use of this barbaric form of safety testing.

First off, the problem with testing on humans is that we somehow have to come up with toxic free controls. That is about as easy as it is to find the Loch Ness monster. Oh wait, there really isn't one, and there is likely no toxic-free individual in our world.

Secondly, what time scale are we using to determine whether a pesticide has a negative side effect? Days, weeks, months, or years? My position is that anything less than multiple generations (four to be exact) is not scientific. The problem of the multigenerational epigenetic effect of toxins is known but impossible to do on humans as four generations will take 70 to 80 years. This is why the effects are tested on animals (another thorny issue I will pass on at the moment).

Third problem arises because of the problem of combinational toxicity. For anyone in the industry to not address the fact that we are living in a world where our exposure is not limited to a small number of toxins is unprofessional. Well, we are testing humans for pesticides so they all have some toxins by you admission Mark, would be a possible argument from the industry, so that negates your complaint. People are different and they live in different environments. To properly test the effects of a pesticide would mean testing millions of people in different locations around the world. Not only economically unfeasible, the moral cost will go up exponentially.

Fourth issue now comes into play. How about the effects on the methylation of DNA in the individual exposed to the pesticide? Oops, not going to be looked at by the industry in this case. And if it is, why do you need to test human beings when you can take their blood and use a micro array? The answer shouldn't surprise you. It will reveal that the pesticides will have devastating effects on the way our genes express themselves. What the bottom line for the future of our species and for that matter all of life on earth is not an experiment I am willing to partake in.

Fifth problem is that even if testing on humans were efficacious we do happen to have a few other species of life here on earth that we share our planet with. Hey, this pesticide is safe for humans but we have some bad news for you, we just killed all the amphibians. Oh well, an economic tradeoff as we do have to save the jobs of those chemical workers whose families depend on that paycheck. And let's not forget the stockholders of the chemical companies. They deserve a return on investment. Please spare me the bull. We have a responsibility to our children and their children not to wipe out life on earth before they come to being. Museums should not be stocked with all those extinct species of animals we killed for no reason except stupidity and greed.

Bottom line here is that there is absolutely no moral or scientific justification for the testing of pesticides on human beings. None whatsoever. To debate the issue is ludicrous and should be dismissed as inhuman and of no real value to mankind.

28. Multiple Sclerosis - A Proposal

"There never comes a point where a theory can be said to be true. The most that one can claim for any theory is that it has shared the successes of all its rivals and that it has passed at least one test which they have failed."

A. J. Ayer

"In order to shake a hypothesis, it is sometimes not necessary to do anything more than push it as far as it will go."

Denis Diderot

"After all, the ultimate goal of research is not objectivity, but truth."

Helene Deutsch

As I mentioned in an earlier chapter, I initially wrote a paper back in 1997 on the relationship between potato intake and multiple sclerosis (MS). While the information and the theory is pure conjecture on my part, I feel that the data I gathered and the observations we made at

Life Balances in Spokane, Washington back in the 80s warranted its inclusion in my book. You may choose to view the proposal with a grain of salt although I would hope that it will stimulate thought and maybe lead to better treatment protocols for multiple sclerosis sufferers.

Multiple sclerosis is a progressive disease of the central nervous system in which patches of the myelin sheath are destroyed. At present, its etiology is unknown despite billions of dollars being spent on research in the past 50 years. The disease causes symptoms such as weakness, visual loss, incoordination, vertigo and incontinence. The symptoms come and go in a series of exasperations and remissions. It usually has a fatal outcome for most individuals within 30 years of the onset of symptoms with a start age between 15 and 50. To a great extent the initial bouts of the disease are mild and the remission stage is lengthy, although there are instances where the disease comes on hard with little remission.

There are a number of theories for the cause of the disease, including genetics, environment, infections, or a combination of the three. The genetic/infectious theory has a great deal of support because of the greater frequency of the disease among close relatives and the fact that the disease is rare among Orientals, even after migration to areas with a high incidence of multiple sclerosis. It has been proposed that MS is a consequence of infection by a common virus such as Human Herpes Virus 6 (HHV6). One of the problems has been finding a viral source to prove the theory.

John Kitkoski made a proposal in the late 1980s. After years of gathering blood test data on MS patients, he proposed that the etiology of the disease is infectious in nature and only attacks certain individuals because of imbalanced chemistry, namely pH, electrolyte imbalances, and biochemical makeup, not genetics. While I firmly believe that genetics may play a role in defining the imbalances of chemistry, we must also look at other nutritional and environmental factors.

The presumed source of the infectious agent he postulated was the lowly potato. A disease known as early blight commonly strikes the potato. Multiple sclerosis is also common in potato growing areas of the world. Furthermore, the disease is most prevalent in those areas that are susceptible to the early blight, although due to modern transportation

226

of foods across geographic lines, this differentiation has been blurred substantially. This then suggests another epidemiological factor in the disease's etiology, the environment.

In a small pilot study conducted in 1988, twelve individuals diagnosed with MS were randomly selected to participate in this study which compared two nutritional/dietary treatment protocols. A comprehensive medical history along with blood test data was gathered on all the selected patients. After six months of assessment, the data was gathered and a correlation analysis was performed. Although no significant correlation was found on the efficacy of the nutritional support protocol given, an interesting bit of information surfaced. In a letter sent to Life Balances from a statistician reviewing the data, it was reported that the relationship between the frequency of eating potatoes and physical changes were highly correlated (-.898, p=<.001). In other words, the more potatoes a person eats, the worse the symptoms of the disease. Correlations to potato intake and mental changes (-.810 p=.004) as well as emotional changes (-.758, p=.011) were also found. When looking at the effectiveness of both nutritional protocols if the patient had a high intake of potatoes, the treatment had a poor outcome. If the reverse was true (low potato intake), the treatment was viewed with positive results. This merits further investigations.

EPIDEMIOLOGY

The most fascinating aspect of the possibility of the potato being the culprit is in the epidemiology. In the 1930s, neurologists in northern Europe reported that MS was more common in northern cities. This gradient by latitude has also been found in the United States and, consistent with the findings, a similar pattern has been found in Australia and New Zealand where the incidence is greater in the southern regions. Migration from high incidence areas to low showed that those who moved before puberty acquired the incidence of the new country. After puberty, the incidence remained what it would have been in the old country. This would back the theory that believes in the presence of an environmental agent. The regional population figures also show unusual numbers of cases in small areas, such as towns in Switzerland and regions of Washington State. When looking at identical twins where one is afflicted with MS, the unaffected twin has a less than 20 percent chance of developing the disease. This supports the concept that although genetic factors may increase the susceptibility of the disease, it may not be sufficient to cause it and more importantly may not be required for its development.

PATHOLOGY

The lesions found in multiple sclerosis consist of scattered areas of destruction of the myelin sheath. Lesions range in size from 1 millimeter to several centimeters in diameter. Most, if not all plaques occur near blood vessels which may indicate a blood borne culprit consistent with the theory of the potato early blight correlation. The potato theory suggests that the virus enters the body during ingestion of the infected tuber and only attacks those individuals with both a genetic and a biochemical makeup that makes them more hospitable to the virus. This occurs during the body's most vulnerable time, puberty. When hormonal development goes on, the postulation is that the body is most susceptible to this foreign invader. It must be pointed out there is some collaborating research done to validate this theory, but there is no contradictory evidence, either.

TREATMENT

In a few cases I have worked with in the past, when the patient eliminated all potato products from the diet, an almost immediate increase in energy was reported, exacerbation periods decreased, and recovery periods increased. This may indicate that the virus may use this particular carbohydrate chain that the potato provides to grow and breed. The theory goes; remove the fuel and weaken the virus. Destroying it from there and repairing the damage is the challenge. It is possible that many of the nutritional and conventional treatments already existing may benefit greatly from the elimination of the potato from the infected patient.

CONCLUSION

It is my hope that in presenting this theory, further research can be initiated which can help patients with this devastating disease. Dramatic results have been seen using the elimination diet along with a balancing of the blood chemistry. Instituting a protocol for following up on the blood test data with an education program on diet, exercise, and stress reduction are important in the successful treatment of MS.

GENETIC TESTING – THE NEW FRONTIER IS READY TODAY

Genetic testing and the interpretation of what all of the different alleles mean is becoming the next growth industry of laboratory testing. This is, in my humble opinion, a terrible mistake. If it were as valuable as some have said, I would be the first to jump on the band wagon. It's not, and it doesn't look like it will be for a few more years (if ever). Before all of you geneticists get up in arms and start throwing evil thoughts my way, let me explain.

In his book, *Biology of Belief*,[122] Dr. Bruce Lipton, an internationally known cell biologist, made a very profound comment when he said, "…we are not victims of our genes, but masters of our fates." What Dr. Lipton is trying to say is that our genes do not necessarily control our lives and health. He comments rather brilliantly that our DNA, while critical in many respects, is also beholden to the environment in which it resides. In many cases, the cellular milieu is *more* important than the genes in the cell. It is well established that genes do not turn themselves on and off. As Lipton further explains, "Something in the environment has to trigger gene activity."

We know that environmental toxins can affect the way genes express themselves not just for one generation but for at least four without exposing the subsequent children to the toxin again. Charles Darwin noted towards the end of his brilliant life that; "In my opinion, the greatest error which I have committed has been not allowing sufficient weight to the direct action of the environment, i.e. food, climate, etc., independently of natural selection… When I wrote the "Origin," and for some years afterwards, I could find little good evidence of the direct action of the environment; now there is a large body of evidence."

Further evidence against the "genes rule the world" theory came out in a landmark paper in the journal *Nature* on April 20th, 2006. Authors Clayton, Lindon, Cloarec, et al, describe the burgeoning field of metabonomics (a.k.a. metabolomics) which shows that environmental factors such as nutritional status, gut microbia, age and disease have a large influence on the way drugs affect the body even in genetically similar lab animals. This is the second time I mention this concept but I feel it is critical in understanding the concept of biochemical individuality. The cornerstone of this article was one line: "The main potential application we envisage for pharmaco-metabonomics is with respect to personalized human healthcare..." They further went on to make two comments, "However, pharmaco-metabonomics has an important theoretical advantage over pharmacogenomics in that it can potentially take account of both genomic and environmental factors..." and "...we envisage that similar methodology could also be applied to predicting individual responses to broader medical, dietary, microbiological or physiological challenges."

What they explained was what I have been working on since 1985. I just did not have a name for it at the time.

29. TIDBITS, TIPS AND OTHER OFF THE CUFF CLINICAL PEARLS

"Information can tell us everything. It has all the answers. But they are answers to questions we have not asked, and which doubtless don't even arise."

Jean Baudrillard

"When action grows unprofitable; gather information, when information grows unprofitable, sleep."

Ursula K. Le Guin

"An old thing becomes new if you detach it from what usually surrounds it."

Robert Bresson

Vinegar and Systolic Hypertension

If you're faced with a high (over 140 mm) systolic (top number) blood pressure, a quick and easy way to help lower it is to use one tablespoon of vinegar in eight ounces of water. This is a safe and effective way to lower blood pressure. Vinegar, a.k.a. acetic acid, combines quite readily with sodium to create sodium acetate which will easily flush out through the urine as long as the kidneys are healthy.

When I was working in Spokane with Life Balances, we had a case where a woman in her 50s was having a horrible time lowering her blood pressure from its normal 180/120. Her physician had tried just about every medication on the market with only limited success. To top it off, all of the meds made her feel awful; this made compliance a major problem.

We recommended that she monitor her blood pressure twice a day and start taking one tablespoon of vinegar in water twice a day without stopping her blood pressure medication. Over a twelve month period, her blood pressure went down to a steady 120/70, her red face disappeared, her energy improved dramatically, and she was completely off her medication.

Gout and Glycine

Gout can be a painful disease and has been known through the ages as a disease of sloth and excess. It is usually marked with pain in the big toe and by excessive uric acid levels. The standard medical treatment is the drug allopurinol. The standard motto when using this drug is that it is one to be used for the rest of your life. Oh, and change your lifestyle and stop eating as much red meat, smoking, or drinking alcohol.

While I whole heartedly agree with the lifestyle change, what I have a problem with is the drug use when there is a pretty simple way of helping alleviate the pain of gout and that is the use of glycine. Not only is it the least expensive amino acid supplement around, it is very safe even in very high doses (not that I would recommend anything over 1 gram a day).

A while back I recommended it to a physician friend of mine for her husband's gout. A few days later I get this fax thanking me for making her husband (and her) happy and pain free. She shared the idea with the local pharmacist and about five other people immediately got relief from taking one gram of this simple amino acid daily.

This little tidbit comes from another book I highly recommend for anyone interested in amino acids; "*The Healing Nutrients Within*"[123] by Dr. Eric Braverman.

URIC ACID AS A MARKER OF OXIDATIVE STRESS

It is now commonly known that uric acid is a peroxynitrite scavenger and as such a major antioxidant.[124] Peroxynitrite is a product of the reaction of nitric oxide with superoxide, which can cause damage to a wide range of biological molecules. What I have seen over the past 20 years of reviewing blood tests, is that the body naturally increases uric acid levels to combat oxidative stress and that gout, especially when the pain begins to affect the big toe, is the body yelling at the individual to give it a hand in fighting oxidative stress.

The first thing I would recommend for someone with elevated uric acid (greater than 5.5 mg/dl) is to increase their intake of antioxidants; especially food based ones like freeze dried acai powder. Decreasing alcohol intake, smoking and excessive red meat is very important as well.

In conjunction with the aforementioned habit and dietary changes, test for environmental toxicity, whether it be heavy metals or solvents as these can increase oxidative stress. If you find that there is toxicity present, all the antioxidants in the world are not going to do much for you.

Elevated uric acid levels have also been seen in humans with high lead levels.[125] For this reason, anyone with an elevated uric acid level or issues with gout should first test for lead (via hair) before undergoing any treatment. If lead is elevated, then a chelation protocol (typically EDTA) may be warranted.

URIC ACID AND MULTIPLE SCLEROSIS

In medicine, it is a rare occurrence that two diseases are mutually exclusive, that is when the existence of one pretty much rules out the existence of the other disease. In the case of gout and multiple sclerosis you have two diseases that do not coexist.[126] While this may not seem important news at first, it may be helpful to health care practitioners when presented with an individual with a potential MS diagnosis. If the uric acid is greater than 5.0, chances are quite slim that they have MS.

How to check your fluid level

My old mentor John Kitkoski had a fantastic way of assessing the fluid level of people who came to him for help. He was pretty adamant about maintaining a proper level of hydration with the caveat that too much fluid was a bad thing as well.

Here is the simple way you can make sure that you're at the right level of fluids for health which in turn will help you keep those ugly toxins on the road to excretion.

First, sit down in a regular dining room like chair. Not a sofa or a barcolounger, a regular upright chair. Put your feet flat on the ground in front of you and place your right hand palm down on you leg as relaxed as possible.

Look at the veins on the back of your right hand. Are they fluffy and sticking up? If not, wait 30 seconds and look again. If they still aren't, get up slowly and START DRINKING SOME FLUIDS!!! No coffee, tea, or sodas folks. Water or diluted juices. Drink a couple of twelve ounce glasses and try again.

If they are sticking up a bit, begin to raise you hand slowly and watch your veins. As you raise your hand there will come a point when they disappear. Note where that level is. If they go away between your chin and eyes, then you are properly hydrated. If they disappear around chest level, you're a quart low. Above your eyes and you are either overly hydrated or you are suffering from hypertension at which point you need to see your doctor.

Epilogue

"Normal life cannot sustain revolutionary attitudes for long."

Milovan Djilas

"We used to think that revolutions are the cause of change. Actually it is the other way around; change prepares the ground for revolution."

Eric Hoffer

"Those who make peaceful revolution impossible will make violent revolution inevitable."

John F. Kennedy

In order to change the way our world views the environment we need to adopt a rule of physics given to us by the great Sir Isaac Newton:

For every action there is an equal and opposite reaction.

When we apply radicalism to our environmentalism we will be met with an equal and opposite reaction against it by those who would oppose change. They will accuse radical environmentalists of being whack jobs and unrealistic. And you know what? They are. We aren't going back to our old Paleolithic, pastoral heritage. So what I have to offer is a social addendum to Newton's third law of physics.

If one's actions are subtle yet profound enough then the reaction doesn't occur until it's too late.

What I'm trying to say is if we rationally discuss making subtle, yet profound changes in our day to day lives and not attack every problem as if it's an immediate life and death struggle, then we will be able to develop a momentum of change that if given enough time, will create enough force to counter any reaction.

Know there are times that radical behavior is necessary. The civil rights movement had its Martin Luther King, Jr. faction of rational radicalism and its Malcolm X faction of pure radicalism. Both were important in making the needed changes occur in our country. Still, each was thoughtful and calculated to induce change. The Black Panthers movement was radical and destructive which caused reactionary responses and delayed the needed societal realignment. This is happening in the environmental movement of the 21st century.

Greenpeace, in my opinion, represents a Malcolm X faction while Nature's Conservancy and the World Wildlife Fund represent the Martin Luther King Jr. faction. All three of them serve the purpose of getting our society to realize what's at stake and are making the changes happen that need to be done. It is the radical and destructive wing of the environmental movement like Earth First! Who drive spikes into trees or bomb research institutes (Earth First! doesn't but others in the movement have) because they disagree with their methods of handling animal rights or environmental issues that create lightening rods for the reactionary right to point at and counter sound policy changes.

If we give the opposition less of an obvious target we can effect more change with greater rapidity than by terrorist activity. The group that tells us to give up everything plastic, stop driving vehicles that use fossil fuels or people who claim that *all* big companies are evil will only get a strong reactionary response which gets us no where.

The ones who espouse rational, easy-to-follow changes in our behaviors will lead us through the narrow corridor in which our world is being funneled through. How much of a strong reaction will you get by asking that everyone change out three incandescent light bulbs for three fluorescent ones? Not much but the impact on our environment and our personal health would be extraordinary.

I'm reminded of a person who claimed that CODEX (an anti-supplement protocol) was coming to America in 2004 and it would take away all of our rights to use nutritional supplements. I fought him and his allies on numerous forums with a rational rebuttal that correctly claiming that this wasn't going to happen and if it did it would be because of a gradual erosion cause by radical "wolf crying" that the radical wing espoused. Instead of freaking out and bugging elected-officials about a non-issue thereby crying wolf when none existed, the more rational method of working towards more effective self-policing of the supplement industry and cracking down on the hucksters and rip-off artists, we would more readily assure ourselves of the "Freedom of Choice" we need and want.

Bottom line is that we need to lead by example in a rational, non-threatening way and incrementally force changes in our society's behavior patterns. We must also be rationally radical when needed to effect immediate change like the removal of thimerasol from vaccines.

Dramatic change can be achieved through small but significant action. This is the only way to give all of us a chance to ACHIEVE VICTORY OVER A TOXIC WORLD.

RESOURCES –
LABORATORIES

METAMETRIX

4855 Peachtree Industrial Blvd, Suite 201
Norcross GA, 30092

Phone	770-446-5483
	800-221-4640
Fax	770-441-2237
Email	inquiries@metametrix.com
Website	http://www.metametrix.com

I credit this lab and some of its incredible people for helping save my daughter's life. Many of their tests are indispensable in developing a foundational base for the achievement of optimal health and protecting oneself from the toxic onslaught of everyday life.

They are known for having an excellent selection of functional tests including Plasma and Urine Amino Acids, Urine Organic Acids,

RBC and Plasma Fatty Acids, IgG and IgE Allergy Panels, Cardiovascular Risk Profile and many others.

Dr. Bralley and his wife Carol, Dr. Richard Lord, Dr. Bob David and Steve Wickham lead a company whose goal is to give health care practitioners the finest tests available, always looking to improve what they have and make a difference in people's lives. An excellent organization with the some of the highest ethical standards in the industry. They will always have a very special place in my heart.

US Biotek

13500 Linden Ave North
Seattle, WA 98133

Phone	206.365.1256 1.877.318.8728 (International)
Fax	206.363.8790
Email	info@usbiotek.com
Website	http://www.usbiotek.com

The dedicated staff at this lab works hard to do accurate assessment of a wide ranging set of lab tests. Their pioneering Environmental Pollutants Biomarker urine test along with the Urinary Organic Acid Markers are invaluable in helping health care practitioners develop potent and efficacious detoxification protocols for their patients.

Their array of IgG allergy tests also are incredibly helpful in determining a full array of offending foods that may be at the root of a number of health disorders.

Doing it right and helping make people healthier is a driving force behind owners Raymond and Margaret Suen's passionate company. I am very proud to have been able to work with them in the past few years.

Doctor's Data, Inc.

P.O. Box 111
West Chicago, Illinois 60186

Phone	800.323.2784 (USA & Canada)
	630.377.8139 (Elsewhere)

Fax   630.587.7860
Email   inquiries@doctorsdata.com
Website   http://www.doctorsdata.com

Focusing on quality and education, Doctor's Data, started in 1972, has a tradition of excellence and ethical standards of business led by Chief Operating Office David Hickok. They are internationally known for their heavy metal testing of hair (Hair Elements), urine, whole blood and red blood cells. They also do a great job at testing for intestinal bugs through their comprehensive stool analysis. After having Dr. David Quig, their Vice President of Scientific Support speak at RenoTahoeFest I, I was impressed by their dedication to science.

Signet Diagnostic Corporation

3555 Fiscal Court Suites 8 & 9
Riviera Beach, FL 33404

Phone   888.669.5327
Phone   561.848.7111
Fax   561.848.6655
http://www.nowleap.com

Their LEAP test is an innovative, patented way to look at the issue of food sensitivities (note I didn't say allergies). It looks at cell mediated responses to 123 different foods and 27 food additives. These responses cause pro-inflammatory chemical releases by our cells.

As you read in Tasya's Story, we credit this test with helping deliver us from her behavioral issues and helping to better control her seizure activity. While it wasn't *the* answer, it was an important answer.

This process seems to be at the root of Irritable Bowel Syndrome (the one with chronic diarrhea) and migraines along with many other related disorders. Their commitment to quality research makes them one of the newer offerings through Crayhon Research and another valuable tool for health care practitioners in the United States.

ZRT Laboratories

8605 SW Creekside Place
Beaverton, OR 97008
Phone: 503-466-2445
Fax: 503-466-1636
Website: www.zrtlab.com

Started by Dr. David Zava, this premier salivary and blood spot hormone testing lab, has developed a series of important tests that do not need blood draws. Research has shown that many of the toxins I wrote about in this book can disrupt hormones (see phthalates and testosterone). Testing many of these hormones can help guide a health care practitioner to develop a truly biochemically individualized protocol to help get the patient back to a level of optimal health.

Crayhon Research offers a combination blood spot (finger prick) and saliva combination test for cardiovascular risk assessment and hormone levels that can be done in the comfort of your home. Having visited their lab, I came away very impressed with their commitment to excellence.

LabCorp of America

31 Primary Testing Locations in the United States

After running over 10,000+ tests through them, I can honestly say I would be happy to run every Comprehensive Blood Chemistry through them without hesitation. With close to 1,000 draw sties throughout the U.S. they are an invaluable asset to any heath care practitioner.

Quest Diagnostics

Numerous Primary Testing Locations in the United States

Like LabCorp, an excellent testing lab for many basic and esoteric tests. Over 200 million tests are run through Quest's labs every year.

RESOURCES – SUPPLEMENT COMPANIES

CRAYHON RESEARCH

5355 Capital Court #101
Reno, Nevada, 89502
Phone   775.823.5333
Fax   775.856.3313
Email   michaelv@crayhon.com
Website   www.crayhonresearch.com

Founded by noted author, clinical nutritionist extraordinaire and good friend Robert Crayhon, Crayhon Research is dedicated to formulating products of the highest quality possible. Michael Vierra, Sue Kopp, and Theresa Edwards are part of an incredible team of people with a simple yet powerful goal to create awareness among health professionals of the clinical effectiveness and scientific evidence supporting nutritional medicine and other natural therapies. Carbon Based Corporation and KTS Products joined with them in August of 2006 to create a truly dynamic company.

Focusing on brain nutrients, these products are available only through health care professionals but its well worth searching for.

The KTS products are predominately formulated by the author of this book, Mark Schauss. Most of the products you will find in their small catalog are unique to the nutritional supplement industry or are vast improvements over other similar items.

A number of the products mentioned in the section about Tasya, are available from Crayhon Research, but only through a licensed health care practitioner. A list of practitioners near you is available from the company.

The company has two flagship products, the first of which is their Peltier™ Electrolytes available in 3 formulas – Executive, Sports and Standard. These electrolytes are extremely versatile and make profound effects on everyone who uses it lifes

The other is My AminoPlex™, the most advanced and comprehensive amino acid blend on the market. The other bonus is that unlike many other amino acid formulas, this one tastes good.

KIRKMAN LABS

6400 SW Rosewood Street
Lake Oswego, Oregon 97035
Phone: Outside Oregon – 800.245.8282
Phone: In Oregon - 503.694.1600
Fax: 503.682.0838
Website: www.kirkmanlabs.com

When it comes to producing nutritional supplements for autistic children, Kirkman has few peers. My ultimate compliment to Kirkman is that I would use just about any of their products with my children, and I do. I trust what comes out of their facility.

Pharmax, LLC

Bellevue, WA 98005
http://www.pharmaxllc.com/index.asp

Created by Dr. Nigel Plummer, the quality of this company's products is top of the line. From probiotics, to fatty acids, minerals to vitamins, they get my recommendation. I use their Four Pillar Daily Supplement as part of my nutritional regime.

Vitamin Research Products

4610 Arrowhead Drive
Carson City, NV 89706 USA
Phone: 800.877.2447
Fax: 800.877.3292
Website: www.vrp.com

VRP has a full line of supplements backed by solid research and reasonable prices. Many of their products are available direct to consumers through their website.

Resources: Websites to visit

Environmental Working Group -

WWW.EWG.ORG

This is the website I most often recommend to people starting their journey into the world of environmental toxicity issues. Run by the Environmental Working Group, this team of scientists, engineers, policy experts, lawyers and computer programmers review numerous papers, policy statements, government proposals and other environmentally related information. They write papers, press releases and lobby Congress to protect people and their health from polluters.

Scorecard.org – WWW.SCORECARD.ORG

The Pollution Information Site is the greeting you get when you hit this site. Find out who is polluting in your neighborhood as well as finding out lots of information about toxins and environmental pollution. If you're interested in your environment, you need to go here.

Earth 911 – WW.EARTH911.ORG/MASTER.ASP

Dynamite website loaded with information about numerous issues regarding our environment.

Children's Health Environmental

Coalition – WWW.CHECBLOG.ORG

One of the richer websites when it comes to environmental toxins, this is a must read for anyone interested in finding out more about the environment and how it affect children's health in particular.

The National Center for Atmospheric

Research – WWW.UCAR.EDU

A great site devoted to the dissemination of environmental effects on weather.

Oceans Alive - WWW.OCEANSALIVE.ORG/

EAT.CFM?SUBNAV=BESTANDWORST

How many times have you been asked "What is the safest fish to eat?" look no further than this excellent site chock full of information of fish safety.

Beyond Pesticides –

WWW.BEYONDPESTICIDES.ORG

An anti-pesticide clearing house of info.

The Collaborative on Health

and the Environment - DATABASE.

HEALTHANDENVIRONMENT.ORG/INTRO.CFM

This website is a veritable treasure trove of information relating health and toxins.

Nutrition Data - <u>WWW.NUTRITIONDATA.</u>
<u>COM/TOOLS/NUTRIENT-SEARCH</u>

Want to find the foods highest in Tryptophan, B6 and Zinc but are low in Glycine, Manganese and Starch? Go here and search to your heart's content.

CDC/NHANES -

<u>WWW.CDC.GOV/NCHS/NHANES.HTM</u>

NHANES is the US government databank known as National Health and Nutrition Examination Survey. Lots of information relating to health and nutrition.

Organic Foods Resource Center -

<u>WWW.ORGANIC-CENTER.ORG/RES.CONSUMER.HTML</u>

Everyday we find more and more information about the benefits of eating organically. This website is a great resource to find out how you and your family can make the switch to organic eating and what the benefits are. Well worth the bookmark.

RESOURCES:
BOOKS AND JOURNALS

BIOLOGY OF BELIEF -
BRUCE LIPTON, PH.D.

Dr. Bruce Lipton, a cell biologist, has written an incredible book about the field of epigenetics and how it affects all of us. Written for both lay persons and professionals in the field of health and science, I highly recommend the book *The Biology of Belief.* If you saw my copy of the book, you would see about 50 flags popping out from the pages and tons of highlighted phrases, comments and quotes.

Here is an example of something I found quite profound (there are hundreds):

"In fact, only 5% of cancer and cardiovascular disease patients can attribute their disease to heredity. [Willett 2002] While the media made a big hoopla over the discovery of BRCA1 and BRCA2 breast cancer genes, they failed to emphasize that ninety-five percent of breast cancers are not due to inherited genes. The malignancies in a significant number of cancer patients are derived from environmentally-induced epigenetic alterations and not defective genes. [Kling 2003; Jones 2001; Seppa 2000; Baylin 1997]"

How may of you have thought that "It's the Gene's Stupid?" when talking about the etiology of disease. Lipton counters with the brilliant comment "It's the Environment Stupid".

The book is insightful, fun to read and a valuable addition to anyone's library.

PLAGUE TIME: THE NEW GERM THEORY OF DISEASE –

PAUL EWALD

Another fabulous book that should be on every health care practitioner's bookshelf and should be read by anyone interested in the causation of disease. It is a must read that will open your eyes about the relationship between infection and diseases like schizophrenia, coronary heart disease, cancer, and much more.

Dr. Paul Ewald writes in an easy to understand and flowing manner which makes this read enjoyable.

OXYGEN – THE MOLECULE THAT MADE THE WORLD –

NICK LANE

If you have an interest in antioxidants, nutrition, aging, science or just want a good book to read, this is it. Author Nick Lane presents a captivating vision of the world in which we live in and how oxygen helped drive evolutionary forces that led to life as we know it. It will make you rethink the way you look at health and illness and give you a deeper insight into how life came about. An absolute must read.

OVERDO$ED AMERICA –

JOHN ABRAMSON

In the summer of 2005, at a conference called Boulderfest, I had the privilage of being on a panel with John Abramson, M.D., author of the book *Overdo$ed America*. His speech ended with a thunderous standing ovation from the room of 250 health care practitioners from around the country. This powerful book uncovers the packs of lies that have been perpetrated by the pharmaceutical industry which has been selling the American public a bill of goods that only helps enrich their pockets yet does little to improve the quality of life.

Every person in this country or any other, that takes prescription drugs should read this book. When they are done, they should buy a second copy for their primary care physician to read. I recommend this book to everyone I work with and at every lecture I give around the world.

THE CONSUMER'S GUIDE TO EFFECTIVE
ENVIRONMENTAL CHOICES –
MICHAEL BROWER AND WARREN LEON

Paper or plastic? Bus or car? Old house or new? Cloth diapers or disposable? How to choose the best options to minimize our affects on our environment. This is a must have, must use book.

ENVIRONMENTAL HEALTH PERSPECTIVES

This government funded peer-reviewed journal and website allows for free access to all their papers and previews upcoming articles before publication. When it comes to the latest in environmental information, this is the place to go to. www.ehponline.org

OUR STOLEN FUTURE –
THEO COLBORN, DIANNE DUMANOSKI, JOHN
PETERSON MYERS

As the New York Times Book Review put it "Its subject is so important and its story so powerful that it deserves to be read by the widest possible audience." This book is as an important as Rachel Carson's "Silent Spring".

ORGANIC HOUSEKEEPING –
ELLEN SANDBECK

A great 400 plus page book on how to save money while doing the right thing environmentally. This book will pay for itself almost immediately.

Precautionary Tools for Reshaping Environmental Policy –

Nancy J. Meyers and Carolyn Raffensperger

A scholarly work that lays out the concept which may yet save our planet and our species. Definitely a book for the serious environmentalist and anyone involved in policy making.

Natural Detoxification –

Jacqueline Krohn and Frances Taylor

A fairly comprehensive book on detoxification protocols. A nice reference book for everyone's personal library.

The End of Food – How the Food Industry is Destroying our Food Supply and What You Can do About It –

Thomas F. Pawlick

A must read if you want to know the truth about our food supply. You will learn how to feed yourself healthier foods and avoid the pitfalls of food shopping.

The Omnivore's Dilemma: A Natural History of Four Meals –

Michael Pollan

Michael Pollan has written what must be categorized as a disturbing book about our food supply in America but one that everyone needs to read. In it he traces how we feed our country and what we really are putting on our plates and into our stomach's. Very revealing and engrossing.

RESOURCES – MISCELLANEOUS

Far Infrared Saunas – The only one I would recommend is the one made by Heavenly Heat. It is my belief that they produce the safest and best FIR around.

> Contact: Bob Morgan, Owner
> Heavenly Heat Saunas
> P.O. Box 2892
> Crested Butte, CO 81224
> Ph: 1-800-697-2862
> Fax: 970-349-6600
>
> www.heavenlyheatsaunas.com

INDEX

N

neurotoxic 28, 127, 170
nutritional supplements 19, 25, 26, 49, 91, 134, 164, 201, 237, 244

O

obesity 87, 109, 110, 111, 113, 121, 264
organic acid test 28, 34, 35, 54, 110
oxidative stress 35, 53, 90, 93, 94, 145, 146, 233

P

parabens 131
PCB 81, 136
pediatric neurologist 19, 29, 40
peroflurocarbons 102
pesticide 28, 29, 101, 139, 222, 223, 248
pesticides 29, 87, 93, 102, 119, 125, 181, 212, 215, 222, 223
Pharmax 33, 62, 245
Phase II detoxification 55, 119
Phase I detoxification 54, 55
Phenobarbital 42, 45, 47, 58, 179
phthalates 76, 81, 82, 83, 84, 86, 87, 101, 102, 103, 134, 135, 190, 196, 202, 242
polychlorinated biphenyls 135
precautionary principle 29, 192
pyroglutamate 54

Q

Quiq, Dr. David 53, 201, 241

R

RDA 91
Rome 69, 71, 207
Rotary xv, xvi

S

Schauss, Dr. Alexander 3, 4, 34

seizure 11, 12, 13, 17, 18, 20, 21, 22, 23, 25, 26, 28, 29, 32, 33, 34, 36, 40, 41, 42, 43, 48, 52, 53, 54, 55, 56, 59, 60, 61, 62, 63, 162, 178, 179, 241
seizures, drop 13, 27, 33, 47, 48
seizures, grand mal 13
seizures, nocturnal 13, 22, 24, 27, 32, 49, 52
silver 52, 53, 69
Skin Deep 104, 131
smoking 90, 91, 120, 122, 144, 149, 152, 189, 232, 233
solvents 28, 68, 76, 90, 102, 103, 110, 121, 138, 146, 200, 233
statin drugs 101, 148
styrene 76, 102, 137, 138, 198
sucralose 27

T

tantrums 48, 52, 59, 62
Tasya viii, xiii, 7, 9, 10, 11, 12, 13, 16, 17, 18, 19, 20, 21, 22, 23, 24, 26, 27, 28, 29, 31, 32, 33, 34, 35, 36, 37, 39, 40, 41, 42, 43, 44, 45, 47, 48, 49, 52, 53, 54, 55, 56, 57, 58, 59, 60, 61, 62, 63, 154, 188, 241, 244
taurine 20, 22, 27, 29, 105
Thames river 70
thimerasol 74, 85, 130, 190, 202, 206, 218, 237
thyroid 112, 125, 132, 133, 135
toluene 28, 55, 102, 138, 139
Topamax 58, 62
toxicity xii, xiv, 25, 26, 29, 51, 53, 63, 67, 68, 73, 74, 76, 79, 81, 83, 84, 85, 86, 87, 89, 90, 94, 95, 97, 107, 109, 110, 112, 113, 114, 131, 144, 167, 170, 181, 189, 195, 202, 207, 222, 233, 247
toxins xiv, 4, 5, 16, 28, 29, 53, 54, 63, 68, 69, 70, 71, 74, 75, 76, 77,

(ENDNOTES)

1. Mirdha, B. (2003). "Status of Toxoplasma gondii infection in the etiology of epilepsy." Journal of Pediatric Neurology 1(2): 95-8.
2. Pollan, M. (2006). The Omnivore's Dillema. New York, Penguin Books p. 221.
3. Hughes, J. (2001). An Environmental History of the World: Humankind's Changing Role in the Community of Life. New York, NY, Routledge, p. 25.
4. Wertime, T. (1983). "The furnace versus the goat: the pyrotechnic industries and Mediterranean deforestation in antiquity." Journal of Field Archaeology 10: 445-52.
5. Culbert, T. (1998). "The New Maya." Archeology 51(5): 48-51.
6. Hughes, J. (2001). An Environmental History of the World: Humankind's Changing Role in the Community of Life. New York, NY, Routledge, p. 74.
7. Shaw, B., Ed. (1981). Climate and History: Studies in Past Climates and Their Impact on Man. Cambridge, Cambridge University Press, p 382.
8. Strabo, Geography, 3.2.8, C147.

9   Hughes, J. (2001). An Environmental History of the World: Humankind's Changing Role in the Community of Life. New York, NY, Routledge, p. 74.

10   Hughes, J., Ed. (1988). Land and Sea: Human Ecology and the Fate of Civilizations. Civilization of the Ancient Mediterranean, Greece and Rome. New York, Charles Scribner's Sons, p 89-133, 125-30.

11   Ponting, C. (1991). A Green History of the World: The Environment and the Collapse of Great Civilizations. New York, NY, Penguin Books, p. 360.

12   Stradling, D. and P. Thorsheim (1999). "The smoke of great cities: British and American efforts to control air pollution, 1860-1914." Environmental History 4(1): 6-31.

13   Ponting, C. (1991). A Green History of the World: The Environment and the Collapse of Great Civilizations. New York, NY, Penguin Books, p. 362.

14   ibid

15   Altug, T. (2003). Introduction to Toxicology and Food. Boca Raton, FL, CRC Press.

16   Body Burden: The Pollution in People. Environmental Working Group, www.ewg.com, 2003.

17   Houlihan, J., T. Kropp, et al. (2005). Body Burden: The Pollution in Newborns. Washington, DC, Environmental Working Group: 76.

18   Cutler, A. H. (1999). Amalgam Illness: Diagnosis and Treatment. Sammamish, WA, Andrew Hall Cutler.

19   Cutler, A. H. (2004). Hair Test Interpretation: Finding Hidden Toxicities. Seattle, WA, Self Published.

20   Benzene, CAS No. 71-43-2: Known to be a Human Carcinogen." Tenth Report on Carcinogens. U.S. Department of Health and Human Services, Public Health Service, National Toxicology Program, December 2002

21   Styrene Chemical Backgrounder. National Safety Council. 1998, www.nsc.org/library/chemical/styrene.htm

22   Di (2-Ethylhexyl) Phthalate Chemical Backgrounder. National Safety Council. 1998 www.nsc.org/ehc/chemical/di(2-eth.htm

23 "Arsenic Compounds." Tenth Report on Carcinogens. U.S. Department of Health and Human Services, Public Health Service, National Toxicology Program, December 2002

24 Dentist the Menace? The Uncontrolled Release of Dental Mercury. Mercury Policy Project, Health Care Without Harm, Sierra Club, et al., June 2002.

25 Reunanen, A., H. Takkunen, et al. (1995). „Body iron stores, dietary iron intake and coronary heart disease mortality." Journal of Internal Medicine 238: 223-230..

26 Salonen, J., K. Nyyssonen, et al. (1992). "High Stored Iron Levels are Associated with Excess Risk of Myocardial Infarction in Eastern Finnish Men." Circulation 86(3): 803-811.

27 Manahan, S. (2003). Toxicological Chemistry and Biochemistry. Boca Raton, FL, Lewis Publishers.

28 Parks, L. G., J. S. Ostby, et al. (2000). "The Plasticizer Diethylhexyl Phthalate Induces Malformations by Decreasing Fetal Testosterone Synthesis during Sexual Differentiation in the Male Rat." Toxicol. Sci. 58(2): 339-349.

29 Geier, M. and D. Geier (2005). "The potential importance of steroids in the treatment of autistic spectrum disorders and other disorders involving mercury toxicity." Medical Hypothesis 64(5): 946-54.

30 Boyd E. Haley's Reply to ADA President regarding autism and Alzheimer's disease linked with dental amalgam. Letter to Congressman Dan Burton (R-Ill)

31 Gordon, C. (2003). "Role of environmental stress in the physiological response to chemical toxicants." Environmental Research 92(1): 1-7.

32 McGovern, V. (2004). "The Stress Factor: Temperature and Toxicity." Environmental Health Perspectives 112(2): 90.

33 Hansell, A., C. Horwell, et al. (2006). "The health hazards of volcanoes and geothermal areas." Occupational and Environmental Medicine 63(2): 149-56.

34 Lane, N. (2003). Oxygen: The Molecule that made the World. Oxford, UK, Oxford University Press.

35 Lane, Nick. (2003). Oxygen: The Molecule that Made the World. Oxford, UK, Oxford University Press, pg 211-2.

36   Anway, M., A. Cupp, et al. (2005). "Epigenetic Transgenerational Actions of Endocrine Disruptors and Male Fertility." Science 308(5727): 1466-9.

37   Lederberg, J. (2001). "The Meaning of Epigenetics." The Scientist 15(18): 6.

38   http://maps.grida.no/go/graphic/mercury_levels_in_indigenous_women

39   http://www.ewg.org/issues/pfcs/20050111/index.php

40   http://www.ewg.org/reports/skindeep2/

41   http://www.awwa.org/communications/waterweek/index.cfm?ArticleID=385

42   http://pubs.acs.org/subscribe/journals/esthag-w/2002/feb/policy/rr_exposure.html Environmental Science and Technology Online News.

43   Tremblay, A., C. Pelletier, et al. (2004). "Thermogenesis and weight loss in obese individuals: a primary association with organochlorine pollution." Int J Obes Relat Metab Disord 28(7): 936-9.

44   Moron, L., J. Pascual, et al. (2004). "Toluene alters appetite, NPY, and galanin immunostaining in the rat hypothalamus." Journal of Neurotoxicology and Teratology 26(2): 195-200.

45   Xia, T., P. Korge, et al. (2004). "Quinones and Aromatic Chemical Compounds in Particulate Matter Induce Mitochondrial Dysfunction: Implications for Ultrafine Particle Toxicity." Environmental Health Persepectives 112(14): 1347-1358.

46   Lee, D., D. Jacobs Jr., et al. (2006). "Could low-level background exposure to persistent organic pollutants contribute to the social burden of type 2 diabetes?" Journal of Epidemiology and Community Health 60: 1006-1008.

47   Wolf, A. and G. Colditz (1998). "Current estimates of the economic cost of obesity in the United States." Obesity Research 6(2): 97-106.

48   Harte J, Holdren C, Schneider R, Shirley C, *Toxics A to Z: A Guide to Everyday Pollution Hazards*, University of California Press, pg 217, 1991.

49 Gamble, M., X. Liu, et al. (2006). "Folate and arsenic metabolism: a double-blind, placebo-controlled folic acid-supplementation trial in Bangladesh." Am J Clin Nutr 84(5): 1093-1101.

50 Poison Playgrounds: Arsenic in Pressure-Treated Wood. Healthy Building Network and Environmental Working Group, May 2001. http://www.ewg.org/reports/poisonedplaygrounds/ch1.html

51 Lasky, T. et al. "Mean Total arsenic Concentrations in Chicken 1989-2000 and Estimated Exposures for Consumers of Chicken." Environmental Health Perspectives, Vol. 112, No. 1 January 2004.

52 Focazio, M.J., et al. "A Retrospective Analysis on the Occurrence of Arsenic in Ground-Water Resources of the United States and Limitations in Drinking-Water-Supply Characterizations," U.S. Geological Survey Water-Resources Investigation Report, No. 99-4279 (1999), p. 21

53 "Arsenic Compounds." Tenth Report on Carcinogens. U.S. Department of Health and Human Services, Public Health Service, National Toxicology Program, December 2002.

54 Drinking Water Standard for Arsenic. U.S. Environmental Protection Agency, Office of Water, January 2001. http://www.epa.gov/safewater/ars/ars_rule_factsheet.html

55 "Arsenic Compounds." Tenth Report on Carcinogens. U.S. Department of Health and Human Services, Public Health Service, National Toxicology Program, December 2002.

56 National Primary Drinking Water Regulations: Consumer Factsheet on Benzene. U.S. Environmental Protection Agency, Office of Water, Ground Water and Drinking Water, Updated April 12, 2001.

57 Benzene, CAS No. 71-43-2: Known to be a Human Carcinogen." Tenth Report on Carcinogens. U.S. Department of Health and Human Services, Public Health Service, National Toxicology Program, December 2002.

58 Ibid.

59 Benzene Chemical Backgrounder. National Safety Council. http://www.nsc.org/library/chemical/benzene.htm

60   Dodds, EC and W Lawson. Molecular structure in relation to oestrogenic activity. Compounds without a phenanthrene nucleus. Proceedings of the Royal Society. London B. 125:222-232, 1938

61   National Research Council. Hormonally Active Agents in the Environment. Washington, D.C.: National Academy Press, 2000.

62   Public Health Statement for Cadmium, CAS# 1306-19-0. Agency for Toxic Substances and Disease Control, July 1999.

63   Lee, D., I. Lee, et al. (2006). "A Strong Dose-Response Relation Between Serum Concentrations of Persistent Organic Pollutants and Diabetes." Diabetes Care 29: 1638-1644.

64   EPA Draft Exposure and Human Health Reassessment of 2,3,7,8-Tetrachlorodibenzo-p-Dioxin (TCDD) and Related Compounds, Part I: Estimating Exposure to Dioxin-Like Compounds. U.S. Environmental Protection Agency, Office of Research and Development.

65   Cory-Slechta, D., M. Virgolini, et al. (2004). "Maternal Stress Modulates the Effects of Developmental Lead Exposure." Environmental Health Persepectives 112(6): 717-730.

66   Screening Young Children for Lead Poisoning: Guidance for State and Local Public Health Officials. U.S. Centers for Disease Control and Prevention, 1997.

67   Report on the National Survey of Lead-Based Paint in Housing, Base Report. U.S. Environmental Protection Agency, Office of Pollution, Prevention and Toxics, April 1995.

68   What Every Parent Should Know About Lead Poisoning in Children. U.S. Centers for Disease Prevention and Control.

69   Jacobs, David E. "The Health Effects of Lead on the Human Body," Lead Perspectives Magazine (November/December 1996)

70   Darbre, P., A. Alljarrah, et al. (2004). "Concentrations of parabens in human breast tumors." Journal of Applied Toxicology 24: 5-13.

71   Harvey, Philip W. "Editorial: Parabens, oestrogenicity, underarm cosmetics and breast cancer: a perspective on a hypothesis." Journal of Applied Toxicology, Vol. 23, No. 5 (September 8, 2003), pp. 285 - 288.

72 Routledge, E.J., et al. "Some Alkyl Hydroxy Benzoate Preservatives (parabens) Are Estrogenic." Toxicology and Applied Pharmacology, Vol. 153, No. 1 (November 1998), pp. 12-19

73 "Chemical Food Preservatives: Propionates and Parabens," Venture: The Newsletter of the New York State Food Venture Center, Vol. 1, No. 3 (Summer 1998).

74 Stehlin, Dori. Cosmetic Safety: More Complex Than at First Blush. U.S. Food and Drug Administration, FDA Consumer, Revised May 1995

75 Manahan, S. E. (2003). Toxicological Chemistry and Biochemistry. Boca Raton, FL, Lewis Publishers, pg. 242.

76 Colborn, T., Dumanoski, D. et al. (1997). Our Stolen Future. New York, NY, Plume.

77 Blount, B., J. Pirkle, et al. (2006). "Urinary Perchlorate and Thyroid Hormone Levels in Adolescent and Adult Men and Women Living in the United States." Environmental Health Perspectives 114(12): 1865-1871.

78 Colborn TE, Clement C. (1992). Chemically Induced Alterations in Sexual and Functional Development: the Wildlife/Human Connection. Princeton, NJ:Princeton Scientific.

79 Houlihan, J., T. Kropp, et al. (2005). Body Burden: The Pollution in Newborns. Washington, DC, Environmental Working Group.

80 Greer MA, Goodman G, Pleus RC, and Greer SE. 2002. Health effects assessment for environmental perchlorate contamination: The dose-response for inhibition of thyroidal radioiodine uptake in humans. Environ. Health Perspect. 110(9): 927.

81 Dahl, R. (2004). "Pechlorate Debate Grows." Environmental Health Perspectives 112(10): A546.

82 Meeker, J., A. Calafat, et al. (2007). "Di(2-ethylhexyl) phthalate metabolites may alter thyroid hormone levels in men." Environmental Health Perspectives 115(7): 1029-34.

83 Stahlhut, R., E. Wijngaarden, et al. (2007). "Concentrations of Urinary Phthalate Metabolites Are Associated with Increased Waist Circumference and Insulin Resistance in Adult U.S. Males." Environmental Health Perspectives 115(6): 876-82.

84 Polychlorinated Biphenyls (PCBs) Update: Impact on Fish
    Advisories. U.S. Environmental Protection Agency, Office of
    Water, September 1999. http://www.epa.gov/ost/fish/chemfacts.
    html

85 Styrene, CASRN: 100-42-5(Human Health Effects). Toxnet
    Hazardous Substances Data Bank, National Library of Medicine,
    Revised November 1, 1994.

86 Harte J, Holdren C, Schneider R, Shirley C, *Toxins A to Z: A
    Guide to Everyday Pollution Hazards*, University of California
    Press, Berkeley, CA 1991, pg. 415.

87 Harte J, Holdren C, Schneider R, Shirley C, *Toxins A to Z: A
    Guide to Everyday Pollution Hazards*, University of California
    Press, Berkeley, CA 1991, pg. 416.

88 Harte J, Holdren C, Schneider R, Shirley C, *Toxins A to Z: A
    Guide to Everyday Pollution Hazards*, University of California
    Press, Berkeley, CA 1991, pgs. 63-64.

89 Ward, H. (1998). "Uric acid as an independent risk factor in the
    treatment of hypertension." Lancet 352(9129): 670-1.

90 Johnson, R. and B. Rideout (2004). "Uric Acid and Diet -
    Insights into the Epidemic of Cardiovascular Disease." New
    England Journal of Medicine 350(11): 1071-1073.

91 Stein, H., A. Hasan, et al. (1976). "Ascorbic acid-induced
    uricosuria. A consequency of megavitamin therapy." Annals of
    Internal Medicine 84(4): 385-8.

92 Braverman, E., C. Pfeiffer, et al. (2003). The Healing Nutrients
    Within. North Bergen, NJ, Basic Health Publications, Inc.

93 Hooper, D. C., S. Spitsin, et al. (1998). "Uric acid, a
    natural scavenger of peroxynitrite, in experimental allergic
    encephalomyelitis and multiple sclerosis. 10.1073 95(2): 675-
    680.

94 Sotgiu, S., M. Pugliatti, et al. (2002). "Serum uric acid and
    multiple sclerosis." Neurological Sciences 23(4): 183-188.

95 Abramson, J. (2005). Overdo$ed America: The Broken Promise
    of American Medicine. New York, NY, Harper Perennial.

96 Ravnskov, U. (2003). "High cholesterol may protect against
    infections and atherosclerosis." Q J Med 96(12): 927-934.

97 Hully, S., J. Walsh, et al. (1992). "Health Policy on Blood Cholesterol: Time to Change Directions." Circulation 86(4): 1026-1029.

98 Krumholz, H., T. Seeman, et al. (1994). "Lack of association between cholesterol and coronary heart disease mortality and morbidity and all-cause mortality in persons older than 70 years." Journal of the American Medical Association 272(17): 1335-1340.

99 Kravitz, R. L., R. M. Epstein, et al. (2005). „Influence of Patients' Requests for Direct-to-Consumer Advertised Antidepressants: A Randomized Controlled Trial" JAMA 293(16): 1995-2002.

100 Mintzes B, Kazanjian A, Bassett A and Lexchin J, "Pills, persuasion and public health policies: Report of an expert survey on direct to consumer advertising of prescription drugs in Canada, the United States and New Zealand", Centre for Health Services and Public Policy, University of British Columbia, 2001.

101 Avorn, J. (2004). Powerful Medicines: The Benefits, Risks, and Costs of Prescription Drugs. New York, Alfred A. Knopf.

102 Group, H. D. T. S. (2002). "Effect of Hypericum perforatum (St John's Wort) in Major Depressive Disorder: A Randomized Controlled Trial." JAMA 287(14): 1807-1814.

103 Angell, M. (2005). The Truth About the Drug Companies: How they deceive us and what to do about it. New York City, Random House.

104 Goozner, M. (2004). The $800 Million Dollar Pill. Berkeley, CA, University of California Press.

105 Rea, P., NFM's Market Overview Research Methodology Explained, The Natural Foods Merchandiser, June 2004.

106 Manahan, S. E. (2003). Toxicological Chemistry and Biochemistry. Boca Raton, FL, Lewis Publishers.

107 Manahan, S. E. (2003). Toxicological Chemistry and Biochemistry. Boca Raton, FL, Lewis Publishers.

108 Bralley, J. and R. Lord (2001). Laboratory Evaluations in Molecular Medicine: Nutrients, Toxicants, and Cell Regulators. Norcross, GA, The Institute for Advances in Molecular Medicine.

109 Clayton, T., J. Lindon, et al. (2006). "Pharmaco-metabonomic phenotyping and personalized drug treatment." Nature 440(20): 1073-1077.

110 Myers, N., C. Raffensperger, et al. (2006). Precautionary Tools for Reshaping Environmental Policy. Cambridge, MA, MIT Press.

111 *Wingspread Statement on the Precautionary Principle*, in Raffensperger and Tickner, *Protecting Public Health and the Environment.* Available at http://www.sehn.org/precaution.

112 Myers, N., C. Raffensperger, et al. (2006). Precautionary Tools for Reshaping Environmental Policy. Cambridge, MA, MIT Press, pg 95.

113 Monbiot, G. "The Fake Persuaders." *The Guardian* (UK), May 14, 2002.

114 Cutler, A. H. (1999). Amalgam Illness: Diagnosis and Treatment. Sammamish, WA, Andrew Hall Cutler, pg. 87.

115 Brower, M. and W. Leon (1999). The Consumer's Guide to Effective Environmental Choices. New York, NY, Three Rivers Press.

116 Powers, RW, "Curbside Recycling: Energy and Environmental Considerations." *Solid Waste Technologies*, (Sept/Oct 1995), 32.

117 Brower, M. and W. Leon (1999). The Consumer's Guide to Effective Environmental Choices: Practical advice from the Union of Concerned Scientists. New York, Three River Press.

118 Harte J, Holdren C, Schneider R, Shirley C, *Toxins A to Z: A Guide to Everyday Pollution Hazards*, University of California Press, Berkeley, CA 1991, pgs. 71-72.

119 Parent Ratings of Behavioral Effects of Biomedical Interventions, Autism Research Institute, 4182 Adams Avenue, San Diego, CA 92116 USA. http://www.autismwebsite.com/ari/treatment/form34q.htm

120 Heritage, J. (2004). "The fate of transgenes in the human gut." Nature Biotechnology 22(2): 170.

121 Netherwood, T., S. Martin-Orne, et al. (2004). "Assessing the survival of transgenic plant DNA in the human gastrointestinal tract." Nature Biotechnology 22(2): 204-9.

[122] Lipton, B. (2005). The Biology of Belief: Unleashing the Power of Consciousness, matter and miracles. Santa Rosa, Ca, Mountain of Love/Elite Books.

[123] Braverman, E., C. Pfeiffer, et al. (2003). The Healing Nutrients Within. North Bergen, NJ, Basic Health Publications, Inc.

[124] Weaver VM, Jaar B, Schwartz BS, Todd AC, Ahn KD, Lee SS, Wen J, Parsons PJ, and Lee BK, Associations among Lead Dose Biomarkers, Uric Acid, and Renal Function in Korean Lead Workers, Environmental Health Prospectives, Vol 113, No. 1, January 2005.

[125] Hooper, D., S. Spitsin, et al. (1998). "Uric acid, a natural scavenger of peroxynitrite, in experimental allergic encephalomyelitis and multiple sclerosis." Proceedings of the National Academy of Science 95(2): 675-680.